Ventilator Graphics

Identifying Patient Ventilator Asynchrony & Optimizing Settings

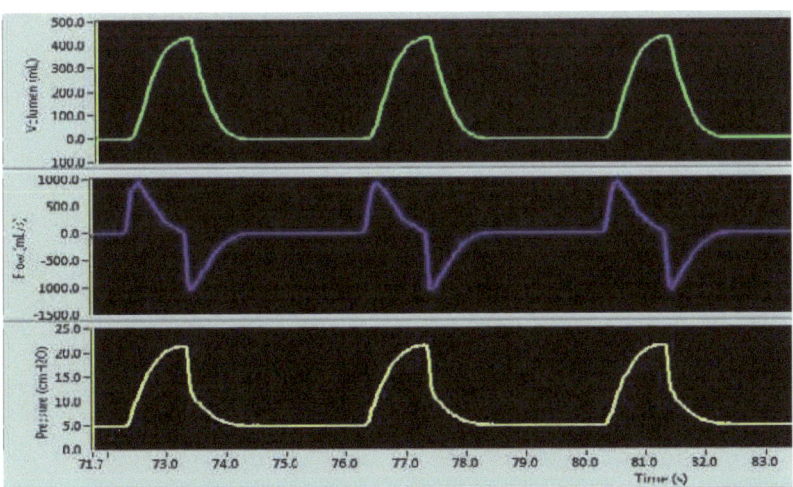

By **K. Scott Richey**

Ventilator Graphics

Identifying Patient Ventilator Asynchrony & Optimizing Settings

K. Scott Richey

Copyright © 2011

Chesapeake, Virginia

Disclosure

All material provided is for informational purposes only. This information is not to replace medical advice offered by physicians, or the medical device operators' manual.

Responsibility of all clinical measures must remain with the device operator.

Preface

This reference has been conceived for the healthcare provider who already has a knowledge of mechanical ventilation & additionally, basic skills for identifying the flow, pressure, and volume waveform scalars.

The purpose of this source is to provide the machine operator with a handy, easy-to-use reference containing primary information in regards to ventilator graphics.

Contents

Phases of the Ventilator Breath Delivery

There are four primary phases in regards to ventilator breath delivery. These are comprised of first the trigger phase, second the flow/inspiratory phase, third the cycling phase and lastly the expiratory phase.

Ventilator asynchronies may occur at any of these stages.

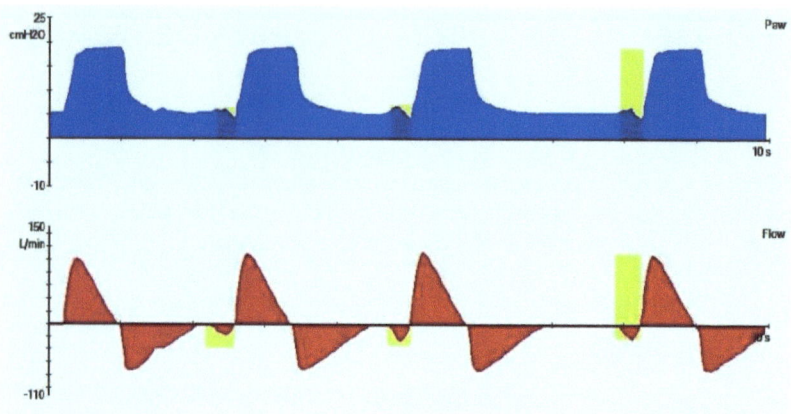

Image 1: The trigger phase, described as the onset of patient effort to the onset of flow delivery.

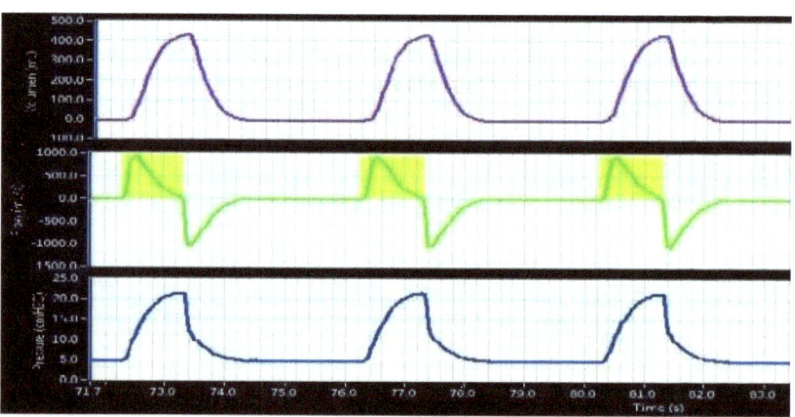

Image 2: The flow/inspiratory phase, described as the onset of flow delivery to the termination of inspiratory flow.

12

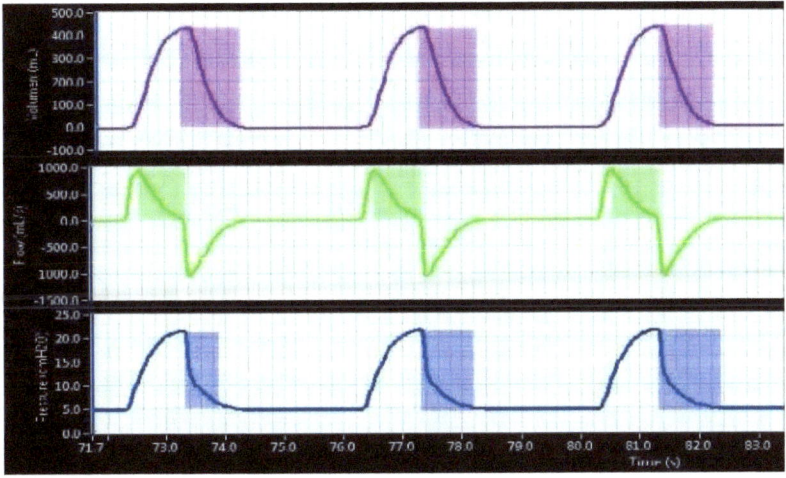

Image 3: The breath termination phase or cycling phase, when the ventilator inspiration ends.

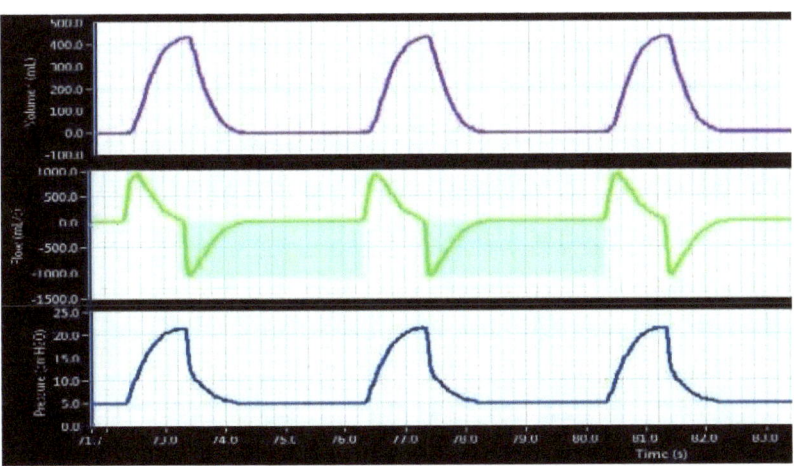

Image 4: The expiratory phase is the relaxation of the respiratory muscles before the next breath is initiated.

Trigger Asynchronies

Optimal Triggering
Auto-Triggering
Trigger Delay
Ineffective Efforts
Double-Triggering
Intrinsic PEEP
Intrinsic Diaphragmatic Rate

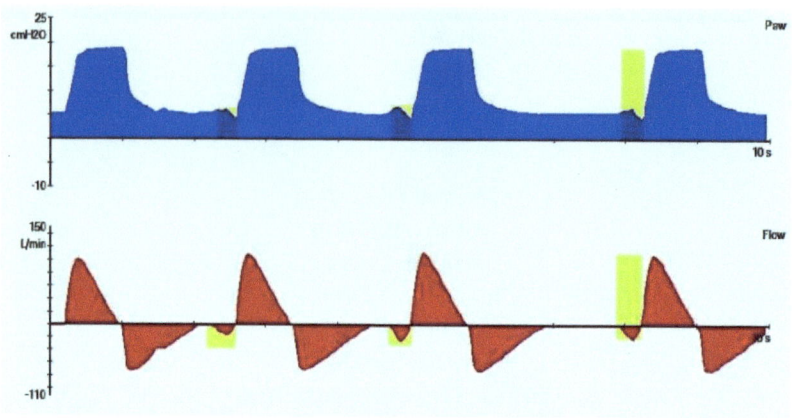

Image 5: The optimal trigger setting. Patient initiated/triggered breaths highlighted in yellow.

Optimal Triggering

During the triggering phase ventilator graphics are used to identify the appropriate trigger/sensitivity setting, trigger delay, ineffective efforts, and auto-triggering. Trigger asynchrony is caused primarily a decreased respiratory drive and/or flow distortions (e.g. ventilator circuit leaks). The above image (image 5) displays an appropriate set trigger demonstrated by an immediate rise in flow following the point of expiratory flow deviation, which signifies the initiation of patient effort. Setting the trigger-sensitivity requires balancing two objectives; to set the trigger as sensitive as possible, so that it triggers with minimal patient effort, yet high enough to prevent auto-triggering.

16

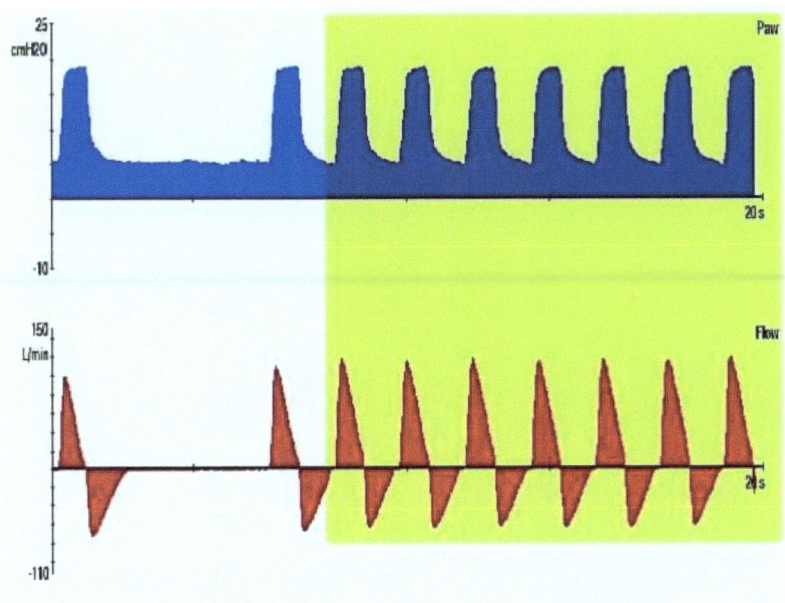

Image 6: An example of auto-triggering high-lighted in yellow.

Auto-Triggering

Auto-triggering sometimes mistakenly referred as "auto-cycling" is a condition when a ventilator breath repeatedly triggers without a patient effort, because the trigger threshold is set too sensitive. Auto-triggering is associated with a low respiratory drive and is caused by various flow distortions; water in the ventilator circuit, leaks (circuit, chest-tubes, and E.T.T. cuffs) and cardiac oscillations (high cardiac output, or balloon pump).

The following breath sequence (images 7-9) shows the progression of auto-triggering after a
ventilator circuit leak.

When analyzing image 9, ventilator leak is obvious by evidence of the volume waveform (green highlighted waveform) never returning to base line. When no leaks are present the volume waveform will return to baseline.

To prevent auto-triggering minimize leaks, or make the trigger threshold less sensitive.

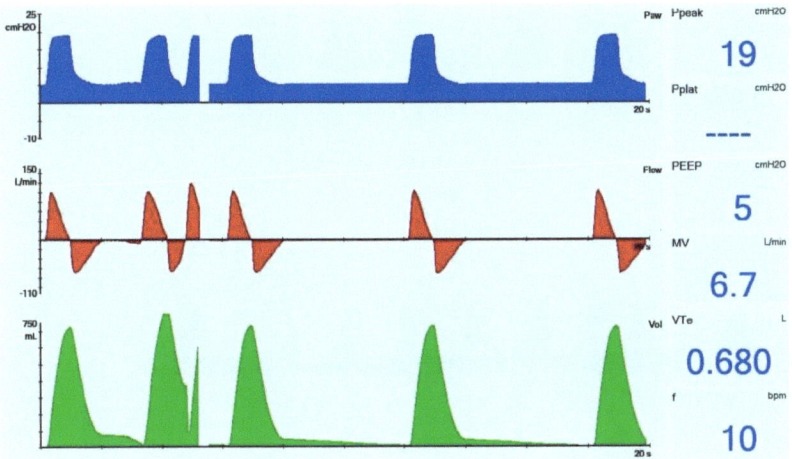

Image 7: The start of auto-triggering.

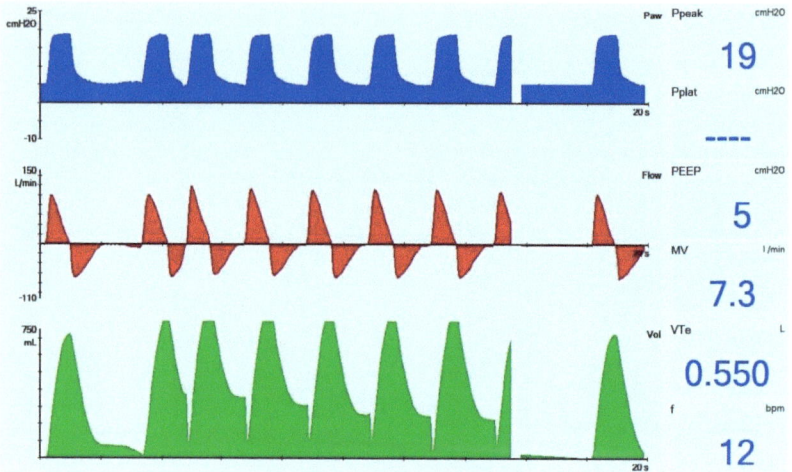

Image 8: Auto-triggering present.

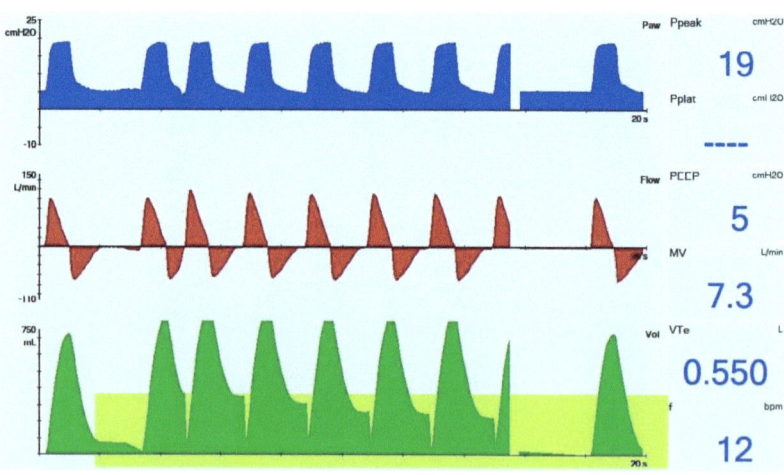

Image 9: Auto-triggering secondary to a leak, by evidence of the volume waveform (green highlighted) not returning to baseline.

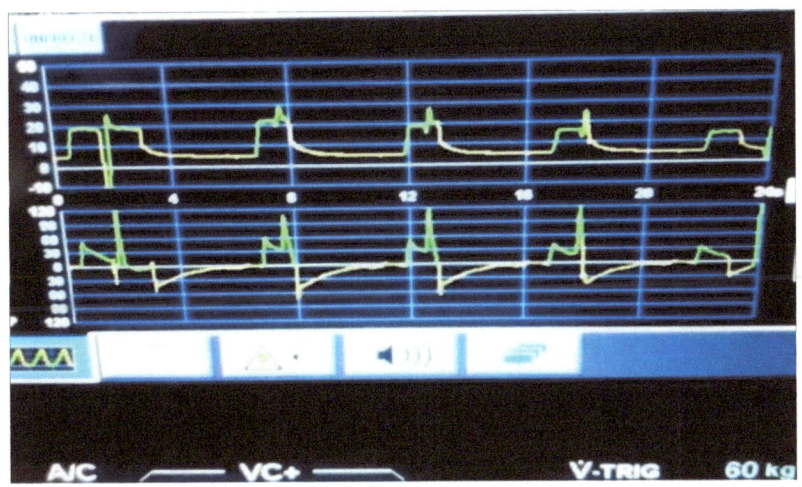

Image 10: Patient with hiccups, however no auto-triggering present.

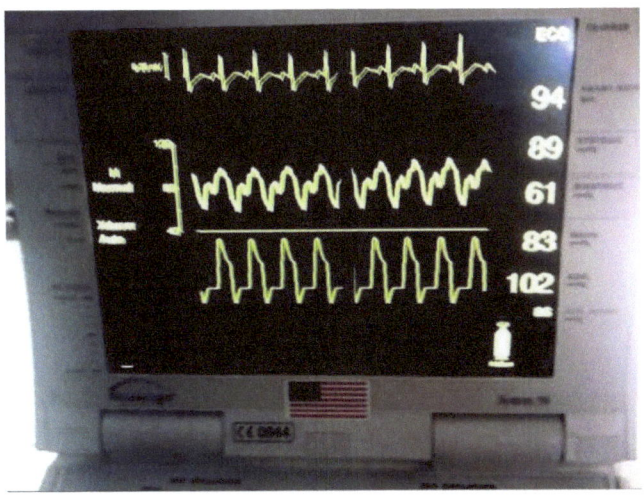

Image 11: Balloon Pump. To determine if the auto-triggering is due to cardiac oscillations consider evaluating the ECG or Spo2 pleth waveform. Does the triggering match the heart rate?

Trigger Delay

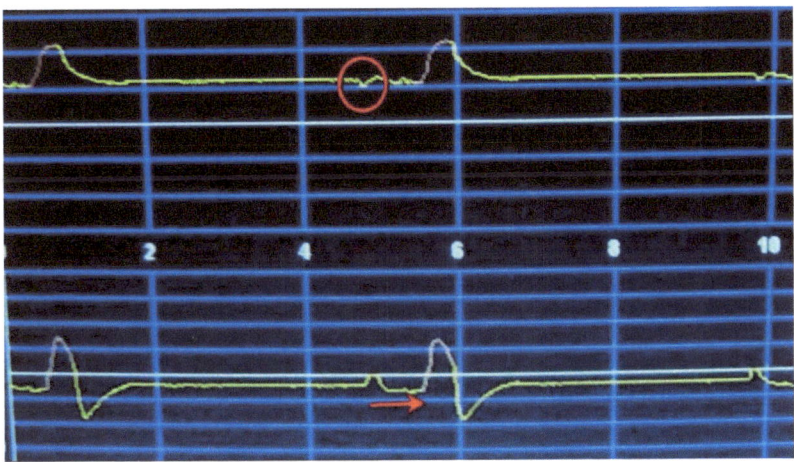

Image 12: Trigger delay represented by the red arrow, showing a latency time before the breath is triggered. The red circle shows a patient initiated effort.

Trigger delay or inspiratory time delay is when there is a lag between the patient effort (pressure or flow deviation) and the rise of inspiratory flow. Trigger delay was common in older ventilators (prior to 2000); however newer ventilators have improved response times. A common cause of trigger delay is the result of a decreased respiratory drive, which may be present during sleep, high levels of assisted mechanical ventilation, hypocapnia, and sedation. The above image shows trigger delay, the "red circle indicates patient effort, and the red arrow demonstrates the lag time before opening of the inspiratory value.

Trigger delay

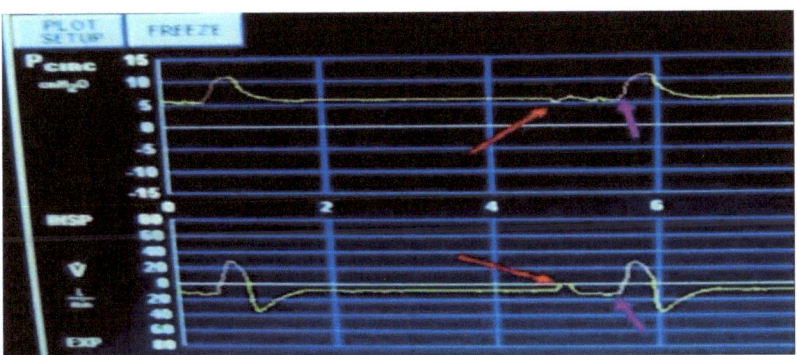

Image 13: Shows a trigger delay of ~ 0.5 seconds on a PB 840 ventilator. This was from an aerosol nebulizer placed in-line, notice the waveform is below the zero (0) baseline. The added flow from external nebulizer sources can cause trigger delays, and apneas.
The patient usually just increases their respiratory drive, and triggering is normal.

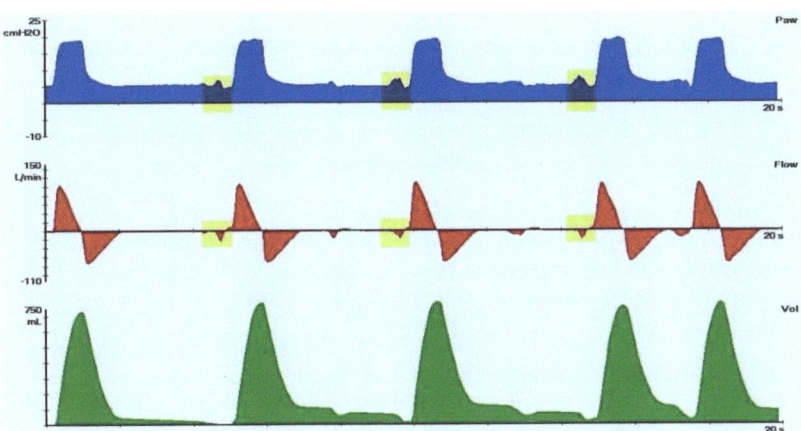

Image 14: Example of trigger delay on a Draeger Evita series ventilator, high-lighted in yellow. The delay is more noticeable when one assesses the "blue" pressure waveform.

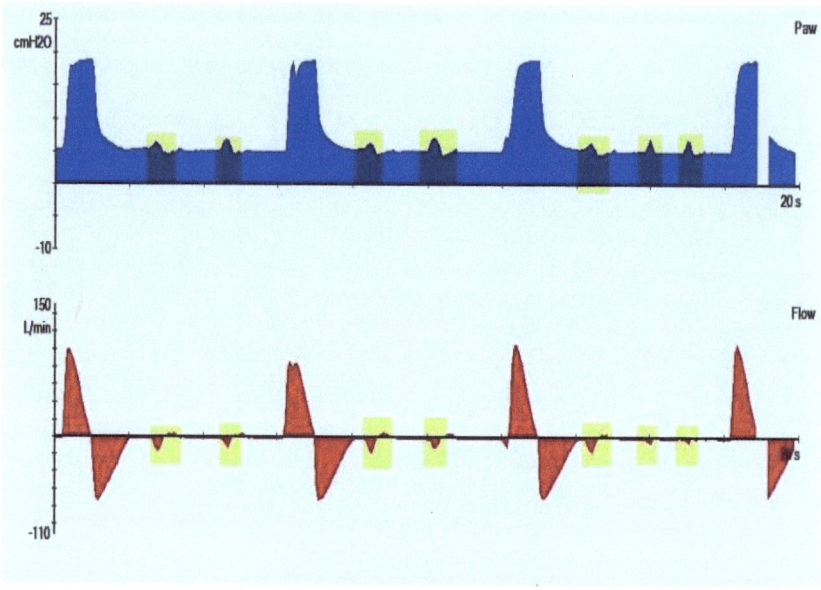

Image 15: Ineffective efforts high-lighted in yellow, notice no machine breath delivered after each patient effort.

Ineffective Efforts

Also known as wasted efforts or missed trigger attempts is defined as "an abrupt airway-pressure decrease of at least 0.5 cmH2O with a simultaneous decrease in expiratory flow that did not result in a patient-triggered breath" [1]. Ineffective efforts are the most common trigger asynchrony and may occur during both inspiration and expiration.

The above image (15) shows abrupt decreases in expiratory flow which are not followed by a mechanical breath, this indicates ineffective efforts. Common causes include; low respiratory drive, and the addition of extra flow to the ventilator circuits during nebulizer treatments.

Ineffective Efforts

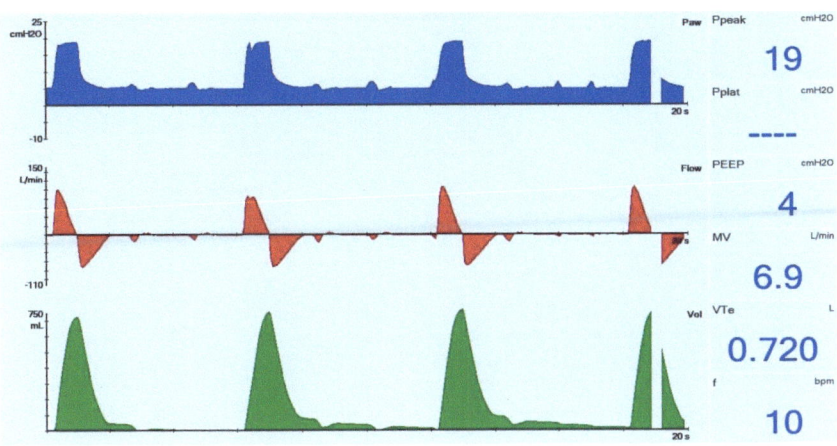

Image 16: Screen shot of a Draeger Evita series ventilator, showing ineffective efforts.

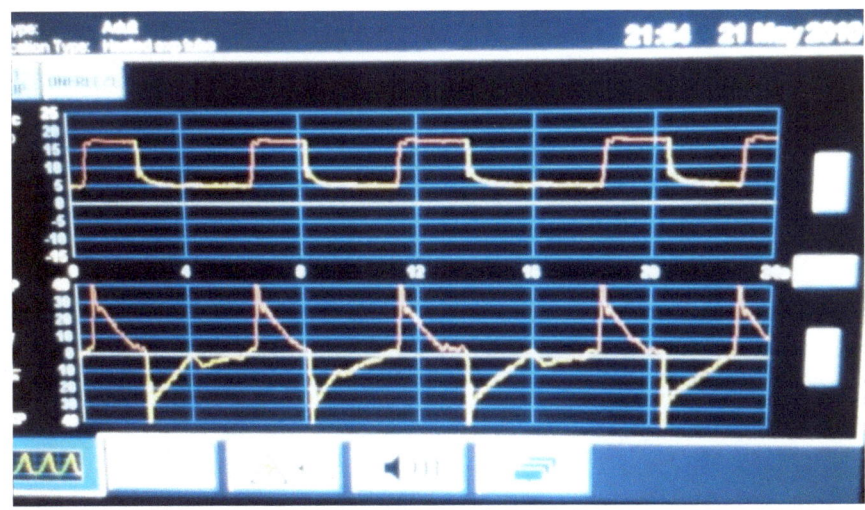

Image 17: Screen shot of a PB840 ventilator, observing the expiratory flow waveform, abrupt decrease in expiratory flow is present without triggering of mechanical breaths, indicating ineffective efforts.

Ineffective Efforts

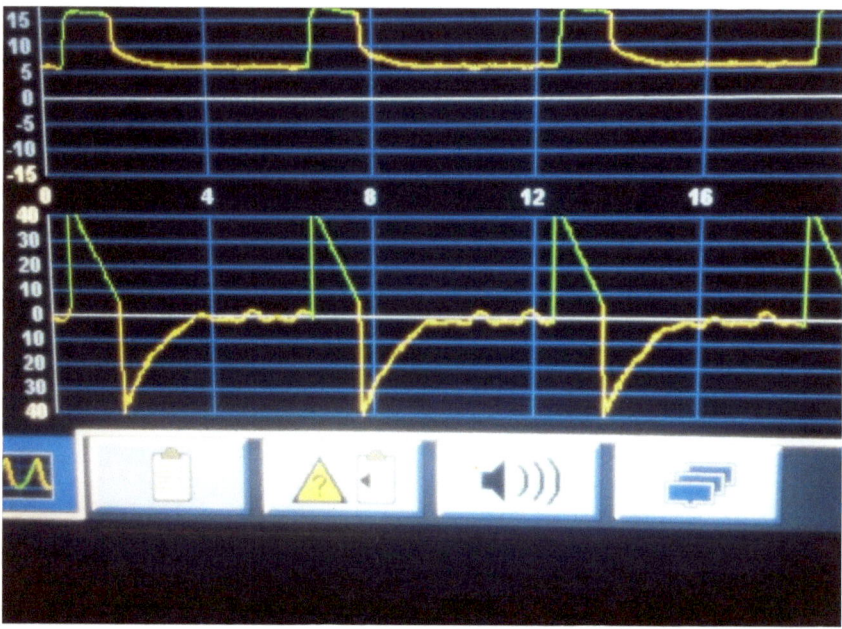

Image 18: Screen *shot* of a PB 840 ventilator, patient has flow distortions due to cardiac oscillations, secondary to a balloon pump.

Cardiac Oscillations

Cardiac oscillations maybe confused with ineffective efforts, particularly if the stroke volume is high.
To distinguish between ineffective efforts and cardiac oscillations, first observe the patients chest and abdomen. Second, place your thumb on the sternum and pinky on the abdomen while looking at ventilator waveforms. If you have efforts without a trigger, this indicates ineffective efforts.

Ineffective Efforts

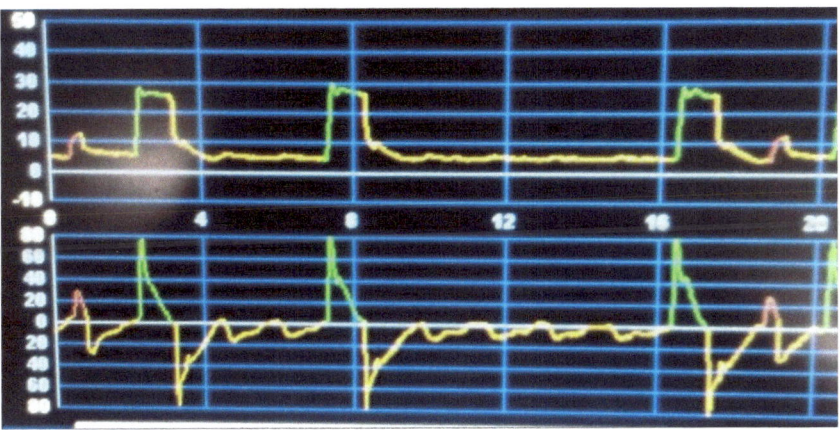

Image 19: Screen shot of PB840, patient with ineffective efforts secondary to aerosol medication nebulizer place in-line. This is common in the PB840, since it does not compensate for external flow sources.

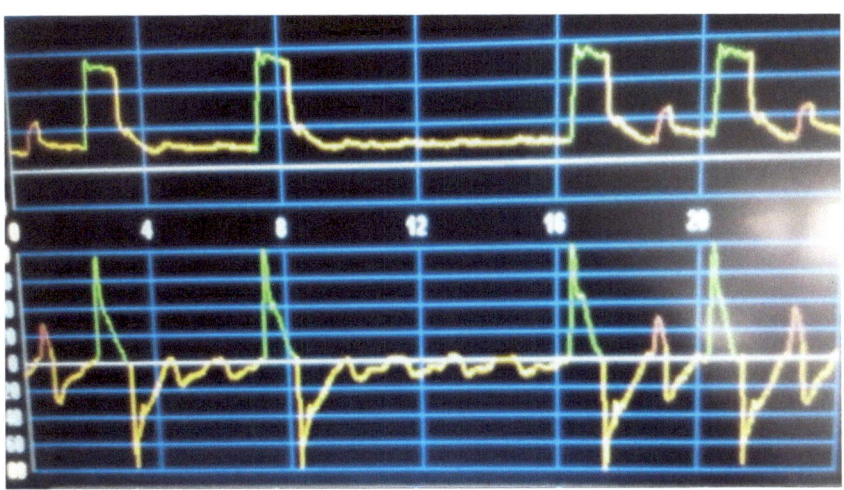

Image 20: Screen shot of PB840, same patient as in image 19; however patients' respiratory drive increased & they were able to trigger breaths.

Ineffective Efforts

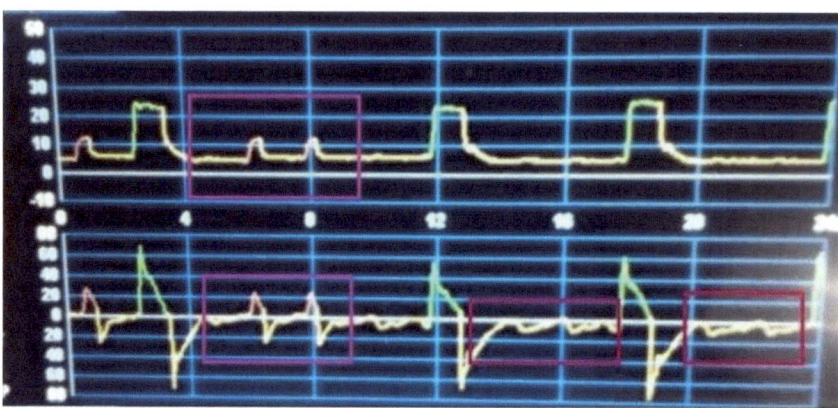

Image 21: Patient was able to trigger SIMV breaths shown by the first set of high-lighted boxes. However, an aerosol treatment was placed in-line (second boxes) and the patient was no longer able to trigger breaths.

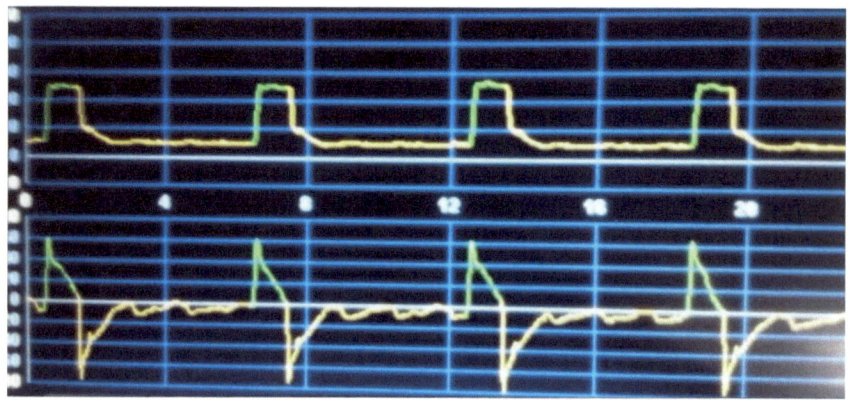

Image 22: Another example of ineffective efforts secondary to an aerosol nebulizer treatment.

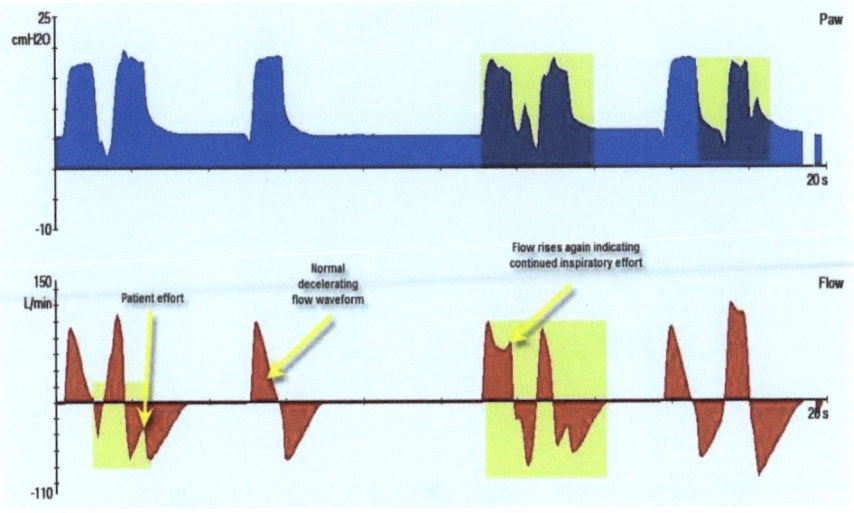

Image 23: Double-Triggering high-lighted in yellow, notice how another breath is initiated before the previous breath has time to end.

Double-Triggering

Defined as "two consecutive patient-triggered breath cycles occur with an interval of less than one-half of the mean inspiratory time (Ti) and is associated with a short mechanical Ti relative to the patient neural Ti "[1].

Double-triggering results from a patient's vigorous inspiratory demand or effort exceeding the volume or flow delivery settings on the ventilator. Conditions that contribute to double-triggering include sighs, coughing, volume or flow parameters set inappropriately low, inadequate sedation, ARDS low tidal volume strategy, high ventilatory demand (increased metabolic rate, high PaCO2, reduced ventilatory assistance).

Double-triggering is not really a problem with the trigger threshold or sensitivity it has more to due with inspiratory flow phase asynchrony, so any effort to reduce double-triggering should focus on the patients' flow delivery to meet patients' demand. The ARDS network protocol directs the clinician to adjust the ventilator or administer sedation when there are three double-triggers within a minute [1].

The following page shows the progression of normal appropriate ventilator triggering to double-triggering (images 24-26).

Double-Trigger

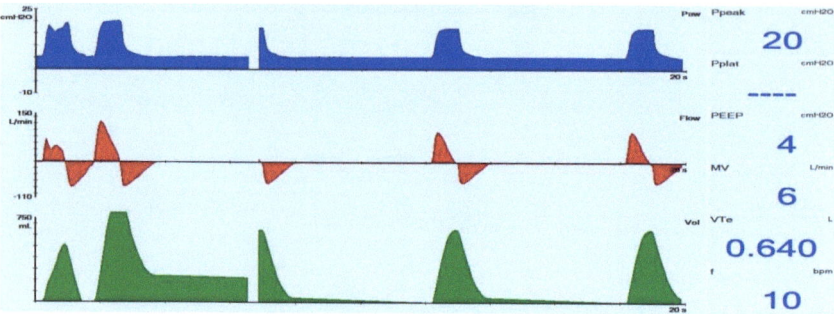

Image 24: One double-trigger present, followed by normal triggering.

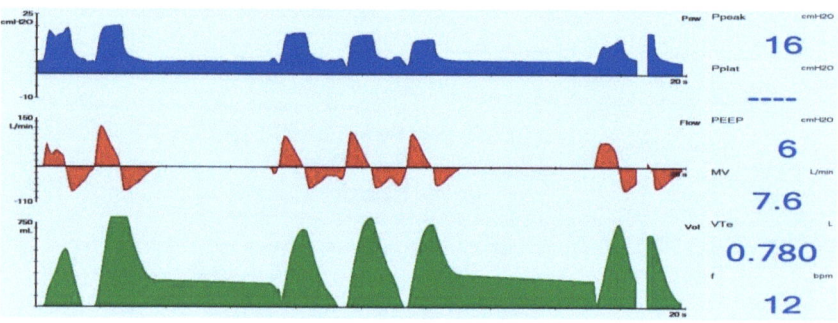

Image 25: A series of double-triggered breaths.

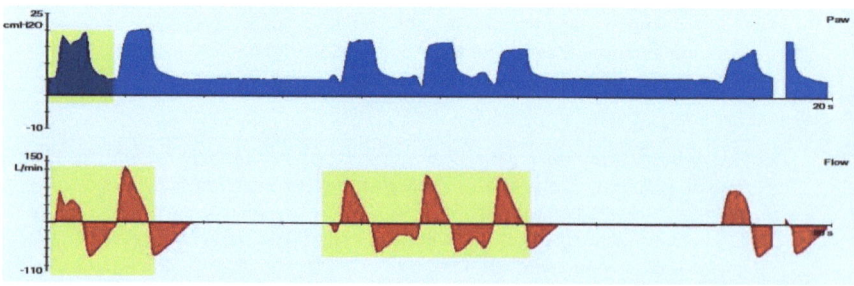

Image 26: The same breath series as image 25, image cropped & high-lighted to show trigger asynchrony.

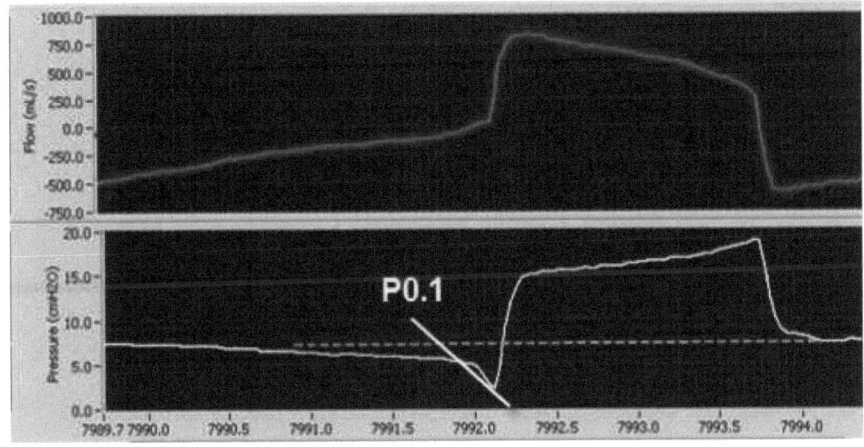

Image 27: P0.1 demonstrated however, the maneuver must be quantified due to the rapid occlusion.

Airway Occlusion at 0.1 Second (P0.1)

The P0.1 is the maximal slope of the airway pressure drop during the first 0.1 second when the airway is occluded. Known as a mechanical index of respiratory drive it correlates with the patient workload of inspiration and may be used to help set trigger sensitivity, flow, pressurization rate, driving pressure, and the amount of pressure support [2].

A low P0.1 (-1 to -2 cmH2O) is associated with a low level of muscular inspiratory activity, which is good in patients with no respiratory disease or damage in the central nervous system in relation to the respiratory muscles.

A low P0.1 may also be due to respiratory center depression (e.g. sedation, overdose, brain trauma/ischemic injury).

A P0.1 from -4 to -5 indicates a larger inspiratory effort, and a P0.1 of < -6 (more negative is associated with excessive workload and/or an increased central inspiratory drive.

Airway Occlusion at 0.1 Second (P0.1)

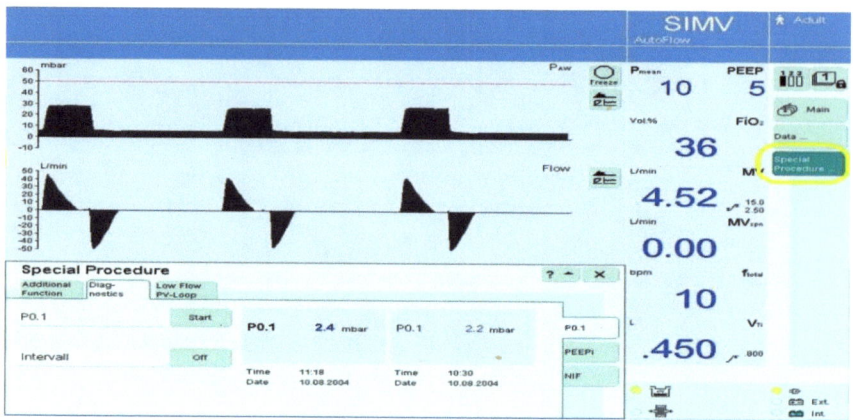

Image 28: P0.1 maneuver on the Draeger Evita XL ventilator, the function is under special procedures.

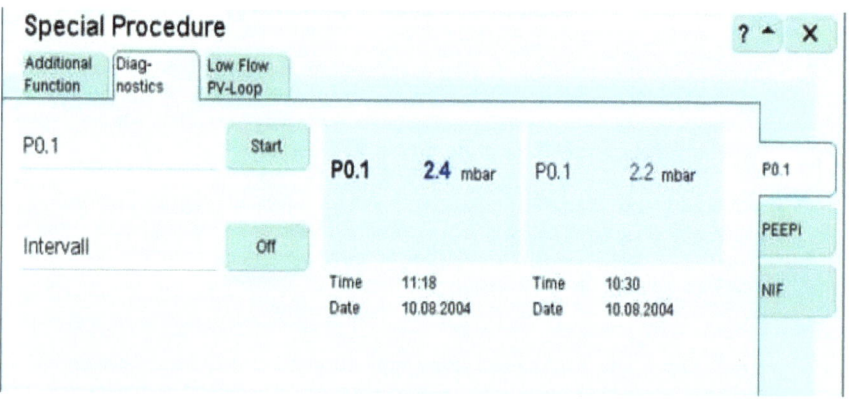

Image 29: The operator can perform the procedure or set an interval for an automated procedure. Setting a time interval is beneficial for trending Reponses to ventilator setting changes.

Airway Occlusion at 0.1 Second (P0.1)

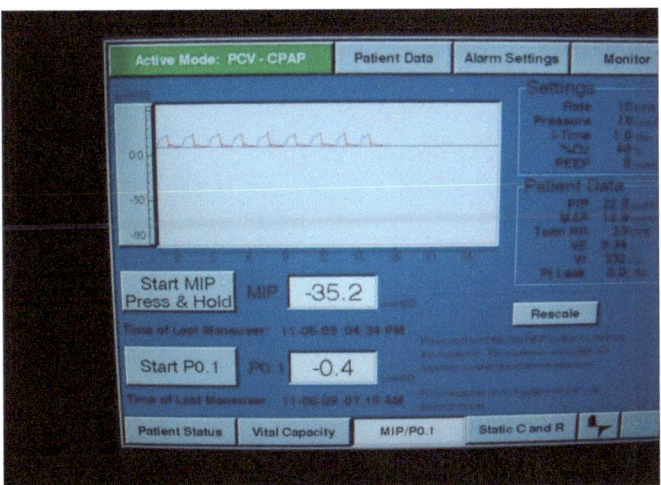

Image 30: P0.1 maneuver on the Respironics Esprit Ventilator, 1st P0.1 -0.4.

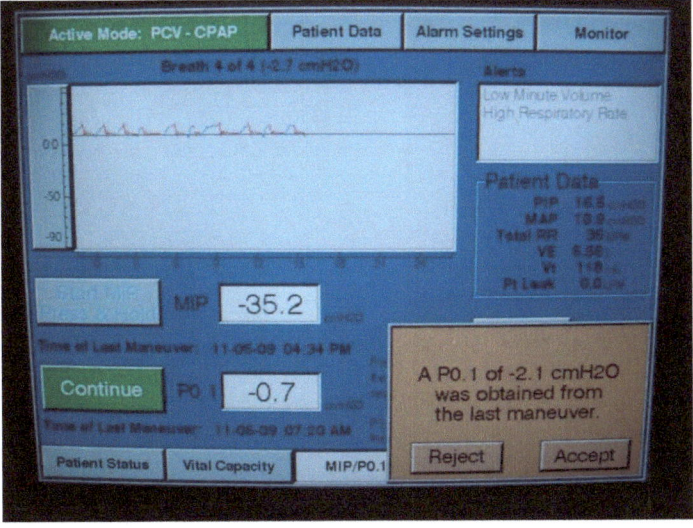

Image 31: A series of P0.1 maneuvers performed for comparison.

Airway Occlusion at 0.1 Second (P0.1)

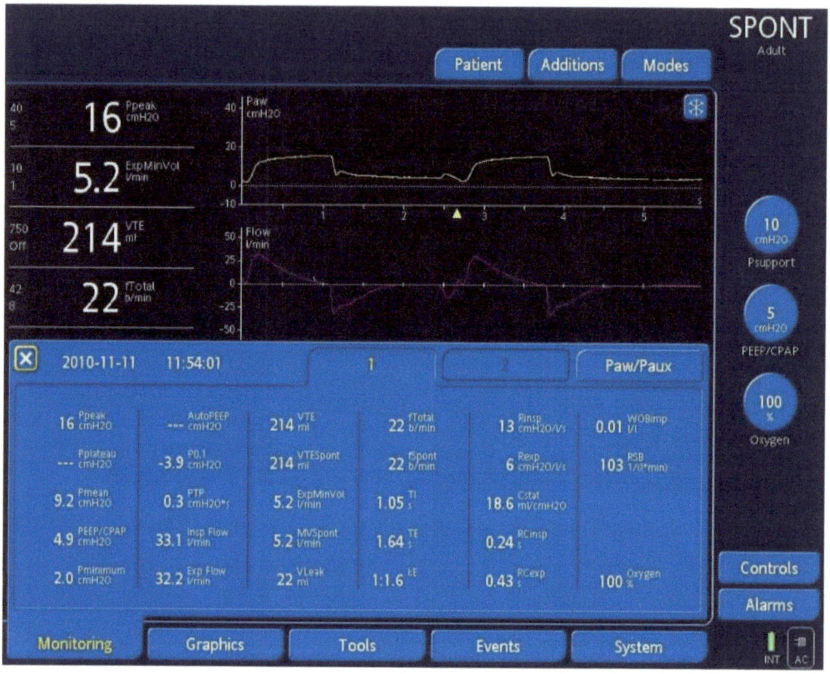

Image 32: Monitoring screen on the Hamilton G5 ventilator, P0.1 is measured continuously.

Note-

Evaluate the P0.1 reading to assess appropriate ventilator settings and evaluate other parameters (e.g. sedation scoring/scales) to assess if P0.1 shows comfort versus respiratory system depression or muscle dysfunction.
Elevated values may indicate inadequate triggering sensitivity, insufficient ventilator support, and that the patient is a high risk for muscle fatigue or failure during spontaneous breathing trials.

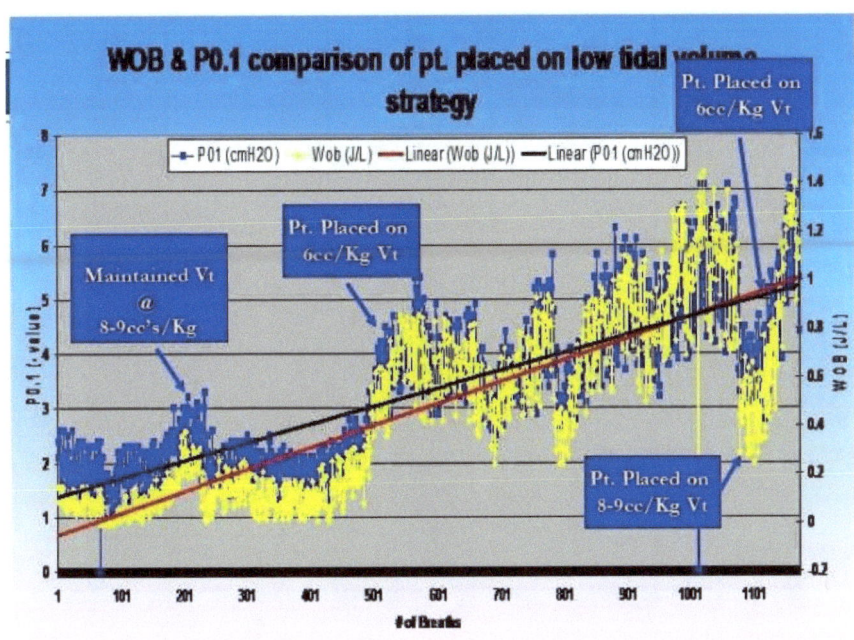

Image 33: P0.1 trending to evaluate patient work of breathing while utilizing a low tidal volume strategy in a patient with normal lung mechanics (grooms, D.).

Clinical Application of P0.1

The P0.1 may be used to evaluate ventilator settings; the above graph provides an example of how P0.1 trending was used to evaluate appropriate target tidal volume settings in a patient with normal pulmonary mechanics (measured plateau pressure, 25 cmH2O).

Notice the dramatic increase in both P0.1 and work of breathing after switching the patient to a low tidal volume strategy (6cc/kg/idbw). Maintaining this strategy would put the patient at risk of muscle fatigue, ventilator asynchronies, increased sedation use, and perhaps prolonged mechanical ventilation.

If the P0.1 is too high (< -5) consider decreasing trigger sensitivity, increase the pressurization rate, increase the inspiratory flow rate, change to a pressure modality, increase driving pressure, or change the mode to Proportional Assist Ventilation or NAVA.

37

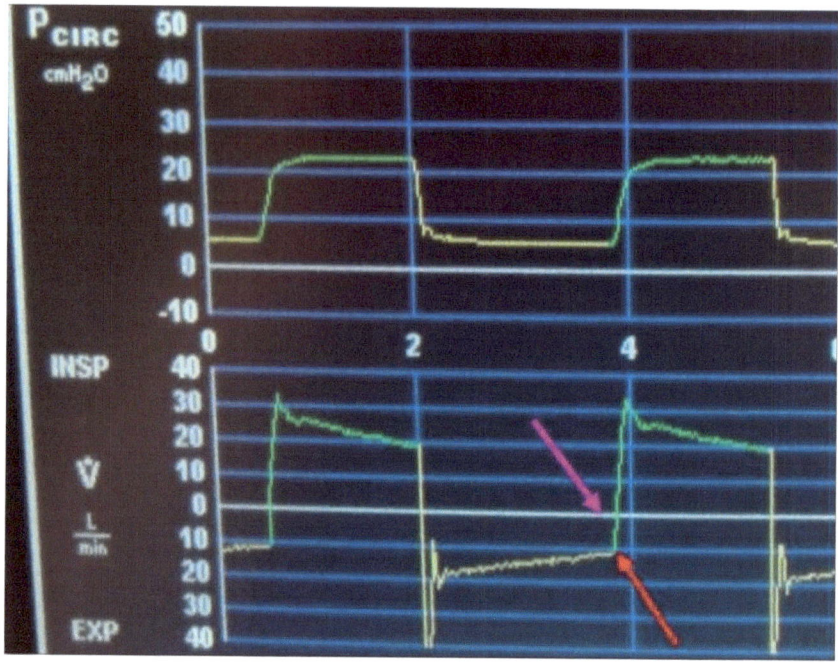

Image 34: Intrinsic PEEP present as indicated by the expiratory flow (red arrow) waveform not returning to baseline (pink arrow).

Intrinsic PEEP (PEEPi)

Intrinsic PEEP also known as auto-PEEP, air-trapping, and dynamic hyper-inflation is actually expiratory asynchrony however, it has an effect on patient triggering and may lead to ineffective efforts. This pressure associated with the trapped volume acts as an inspiratory threshold load to be overcome by the patient during spontaneous breathing.

Increased risks of PEEPi include a minute ventilation > 15 lpm, airway resistance > 15 cmH2O, and evidence of expiratory flow obstruction. The above image shows evidence of expiratory flow obstruction easily identified by the expiratory flow waveform not returning to baseline.

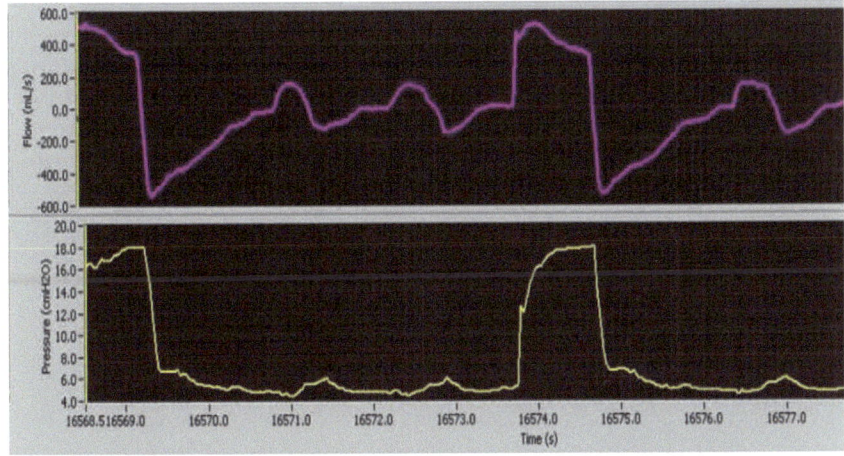

Image 35: Missed trigger attempts, notice the flow distortions (purple flow waveform) without associated breaths. Ventilator measured rate 12 bpm; however true intrinsic rate 30 bpm.

Intrinsic Diaphragmatic Rate

Many patients receiving mechanical ventilation have high intrinsic diaphragmatic rates (≥30 breaths per minute) even when very well assisted [3]. This is usually unnoticed because the ventilator only measures machine or patient triggered breaths; however the patient's true respiratory rate may be higher. This can be problematic when performing a spontaneous breathing trial (SBT) for a couple of reasons.

First, a number of institutions perform SBT's while the patient is still hooked to the ventilator. The ventilator will not detect the ineffective efforts so when calculating the frequency/tidal volume (F/VT) based on the ventilators measured total frequency one may obtain a false positive. Example a patient's measured Vt is 300 ml & true intrinsic rate is 35 bpm however, the machine only measures 30, so your calculated f/vt equals 100 when it is actually 116.

Intrinsic Diaphragmatic Rate

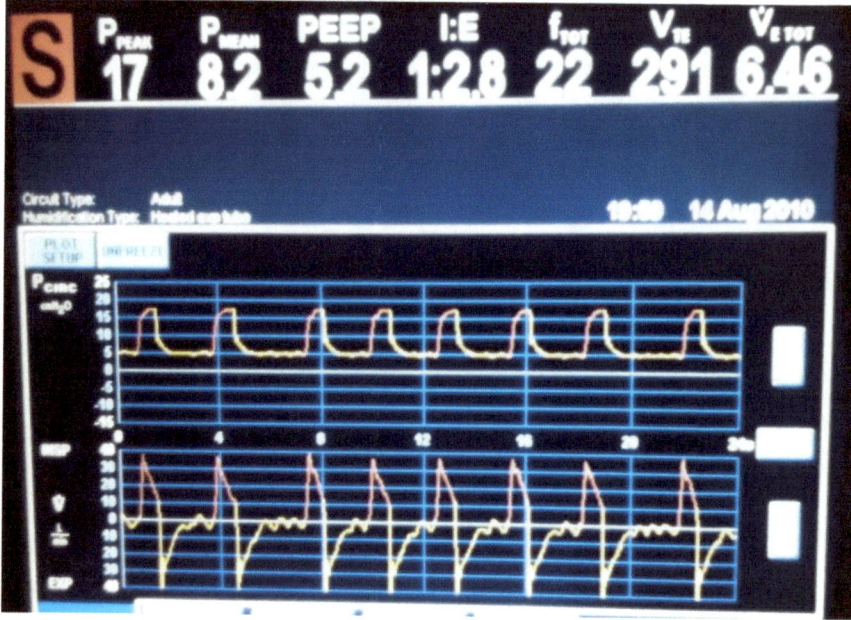

Image 36: PS 12 cmH2O measured rate 22 however intrinsic rate > 30, notice the flow distortions indicating ineffective efforts.

Second, when the operator decreases the level of assist the measured respiratory rate may immediately increase. This immediate increase in respiratory rate is not distress, what is happening is there is less dynamic hyper-inflation due to the reduction in pressure support. So the ineffective efforts are eliminated and the intrinsic rate is captured. These sudden increases in respiratory rate may lead the operator to think that the patient is in distress. This may result in placing the patient on a higher level of assist and prolonging the weaning process.

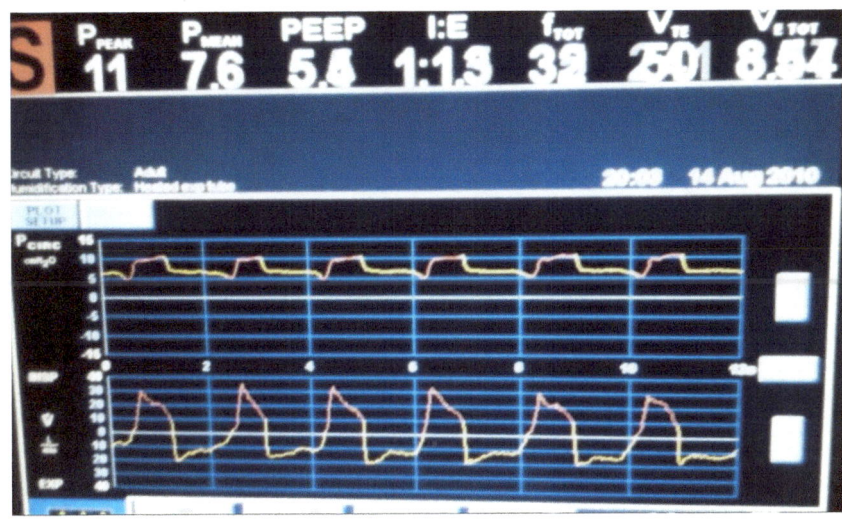

Image 37: Same patient as image 36, pressure support decreased to 7 cmH2O and total frequency went from 22 to 32. However, no ineffective efforts present all breaths have been captured.

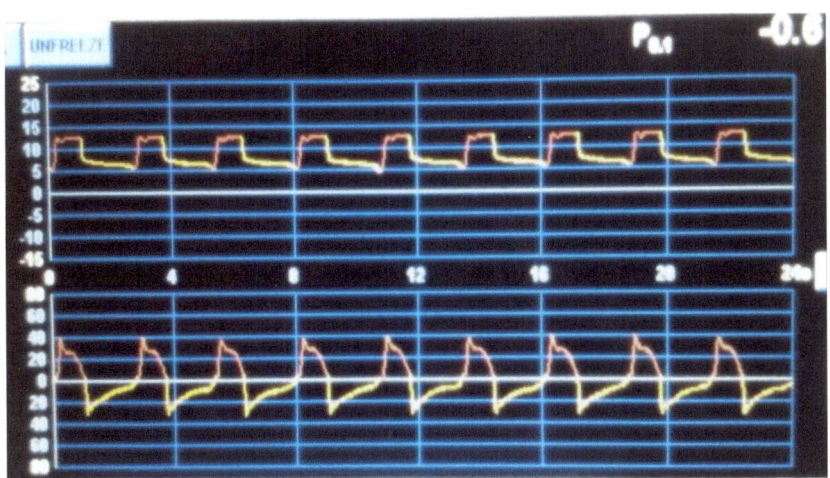

Image 38: Same patient as in previous images (36, 37) patient has a high measured frequency but is not in distress. A P0.1 maneuver was performed with a measured value of – 0.6 indicating no distress present.

Trigger Asynchronies

Conclusion

During the triggering phase strategies for preventing asynchronies include measures that decrease PEEPi, increase respiratory drive, and/or reducing the use of sedation. The operator may consider counter balancing PEEPi with circuit PEEP, increasing the set PEEP by 1-2 cmH2O increments while assessing if triggering improves. Usually no more than 8 cmH2O of PEEP is needed or increase PEEP until peak pressures increase (VC-CMV) or tidal volume drops (PC-CMV).
If available the operator may consider using Neurally Adjusted Ventilatory Assist (NAVA), which triggers the breath based on diaphragmatic EMG signal versus the traditional flow or pressure trigger.

Flow Asynchronies

Flow Mismatch
Driving Pressure
Pressurization Rate

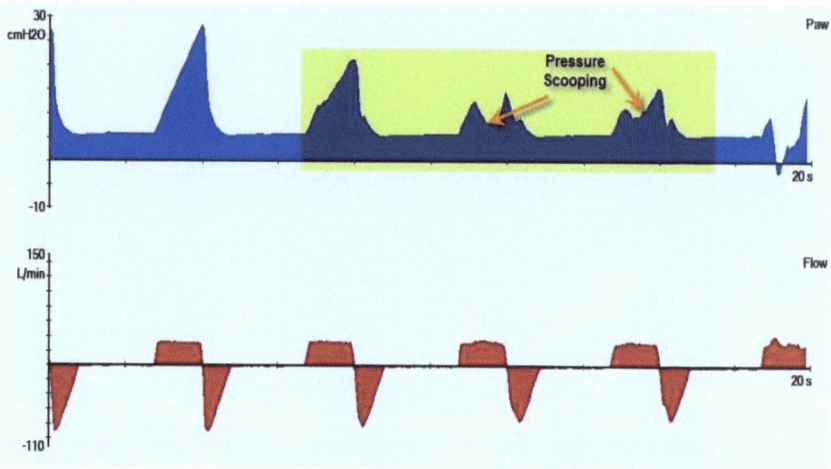

Image 39: Flow mismatch *as* evidence by the scooping in the pressure (blue) waveform, high-lighted.

Flow Mismatch

A common flow asynchrony associated with volume ventilation is "flow Mismatch". Flow mismatch results when the patient's respiratory drive increases and the fixed/set flow rate cannot provide enough assist to meet the patient's demand. This can be present in patients with a high metabolic demand (e.g. burns, sepsis, and fever), patients ventilated with a low tidal volume strategy (4-6 ml/kg), agitation; due to pain or substance abuse withdraw ICU psychosis, sleep deprivation, or anxiety, and during sleep wake cycles.

Flow mismatch is easy to identify from ventilator waveform analysis. When utilizing volume ventilation evaluate the pressure waveform, this will provide the most information in regards to changes in lung mechanics, appropriate flow setting, patient effort, and synchrony.

Flow mismatch is identified by 'pressure scooping' in the pressure waveform. Flow mismatch may be present during any part of the inspiratory phase, the above image demonstrates flow mismatch during the middle of the inspiratory flow phase or mid-inspiratory flow. Additionally, the operator can monitor the P0.1 to quantify excessive effort.
The following two images (38, 39) shows flow synchrony progression to flow mismatch as the patients inspiratory drive increases.

44

Flow Mismatch

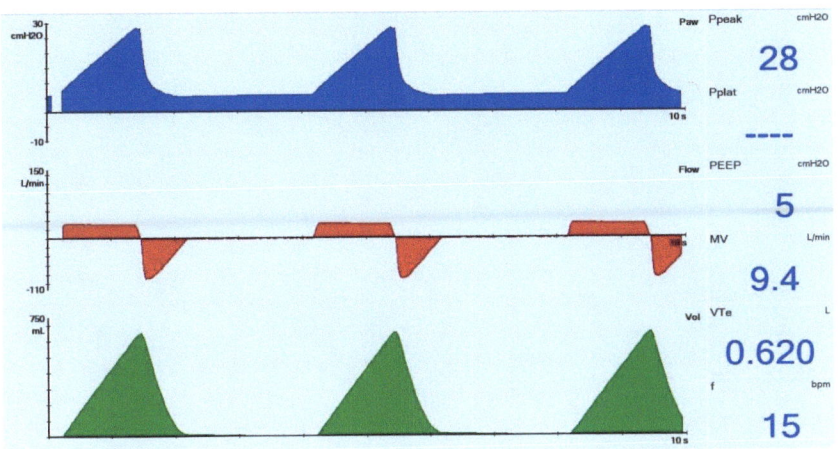

Image 40: Flow synchrony during VC-CMV, notice the regular pressure (blue) waveform.

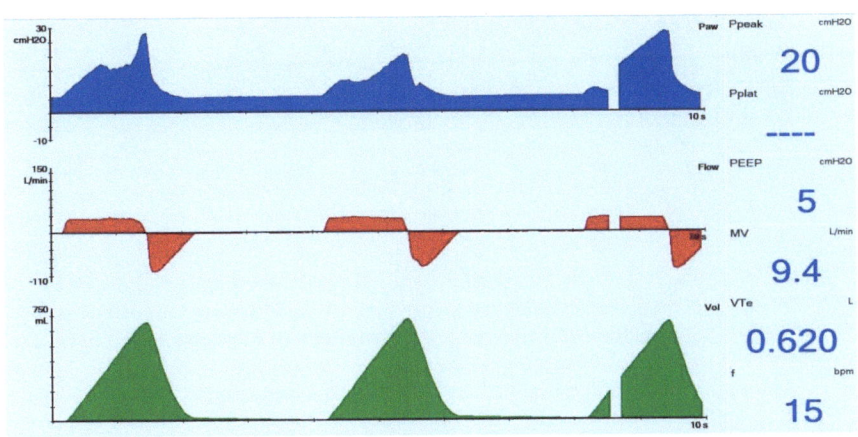

Image 41: Flow asynchrony during VC-CMV, as evidence from the scooping pressure waveform.

Flow Mismatch

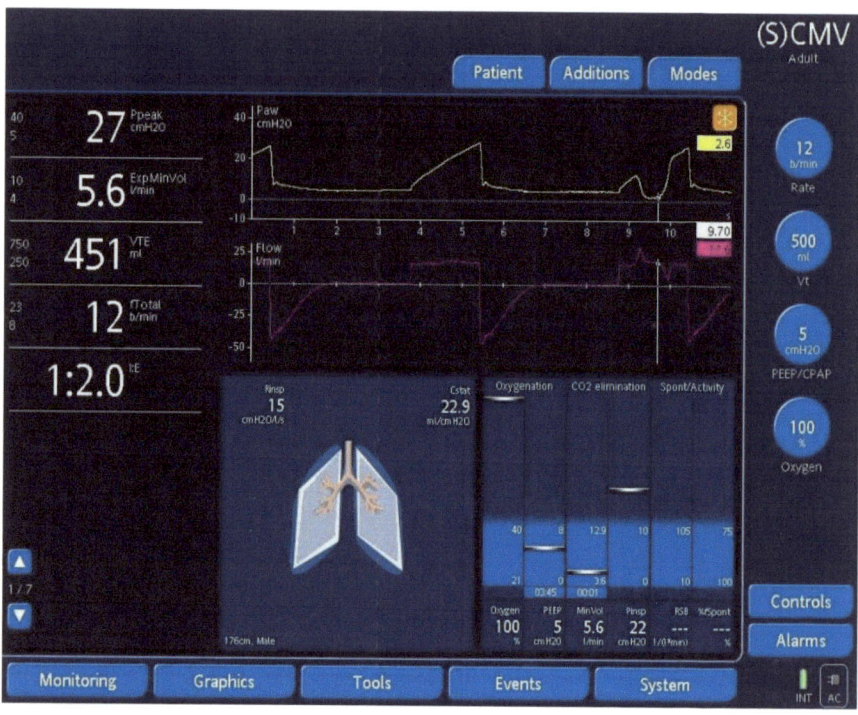

Image 42: Mid-inspiratory flow mismatch, notice the pressure scooping on the yellow pressure waveform, also the measured pressure during the scooping is 2.6 cmH2O, much different from the previous peak pressure of 27 cmH2O.

To correct flow mismatch titrate the flow rate to match the patient's inspiratory demands. Another corrective action is switching from a constant flow pattern to a decelerating flow pattern; this provides a high initial peak flow.

One must consider that changes in ventilatory demand may result in unnecessary higher than average assist resulting in ventilator induced diaphragm dysfunction [7, 8], a lower PaCO2 set-point, and delay in liberation.

Flow Mismatch

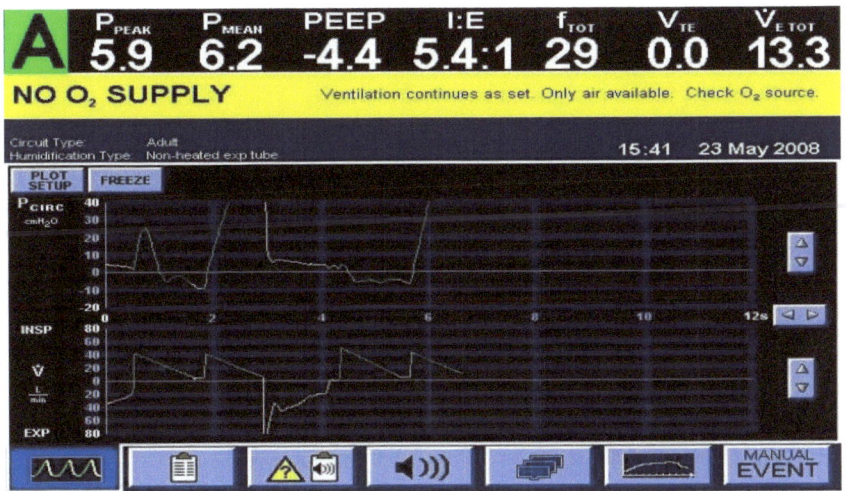

Image 43: Another sign of flow mismatch is from the measured peak pressure reading, notice that the peak pressure is only 5.9 cmH2O & the PEEP is -4.4, this patient has an extreme inspiratory demand.

To prevent flow mismatch consider using pressure control based modalities (e.g. PC-CMV, PC-CSV, Adaptive Pressure Control) this allows for the inspiratory flow to increase automatically during changing ventilatory demands.

Basic pressure modes do allow for the patient to receive inspiratory flow based on their demand however, these modes may not unload ventilatory muscles sufficiently in patients with compromised lung mechanics (e.g. ARDS). When comparing VC-CMV to PC-CMV and adaptive Pressure control the pressure modalities provided no advantage over VC-CMV with a high peak flow rate [9].

Another consideration is utilizing advance pressure based modes (PAV, NAVA) which provide both unlimited inspiratory flow and decrease work of breathing by providing assistance proportional to the patients demand (PAV) or relative assistance to the demand detected by a neural signal (NAVA).

Flow Mismatch

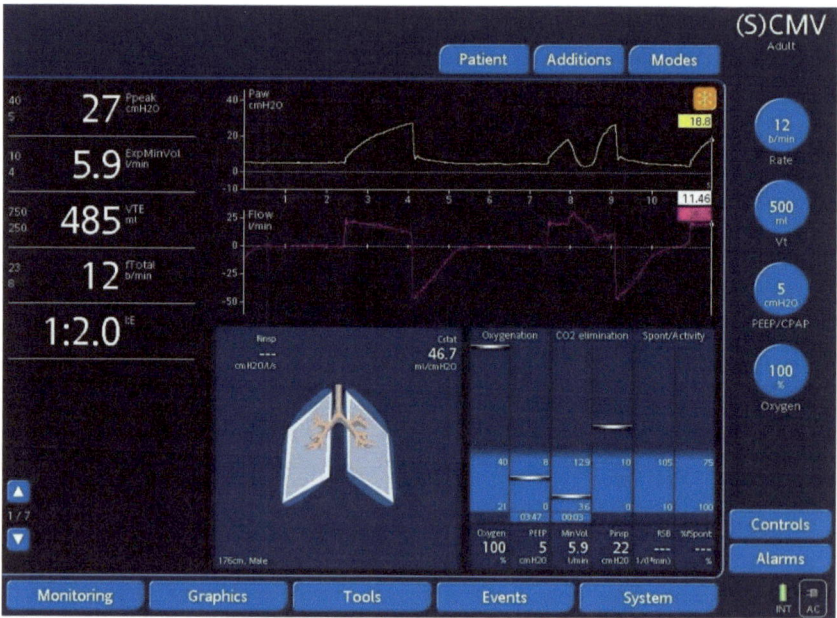

Image 44: Another example of flow mismatch.

Adaptive Support Ventilation may also be considered, this advance pressure based mode utilizes the least work of breathing equation to determine frequency and tidal volume. Furthermore the operator can adjust the percent minute ventilation setting to allow for additional ventilator assistance during periods of increased respiratory demand.
Lastly, consider increasing sedation if the patient's ventilatory demand and/or tidal volume exceed clinical goals.

Flow mismatch is a common patient ventilatory asynchrony associated with volume ventilation. Flow mismatch may lead to cardiovascular instability, increased oxygen consumption, increased carbon dioxide production, increased patient discomfort and prolonged mechanical ventilation [4].

Fortunately, flow mismatch can be simply identified with the proper assessment of the pressure waveform, and can be prevented by utilizing pressure based ventilatory modalities [5].

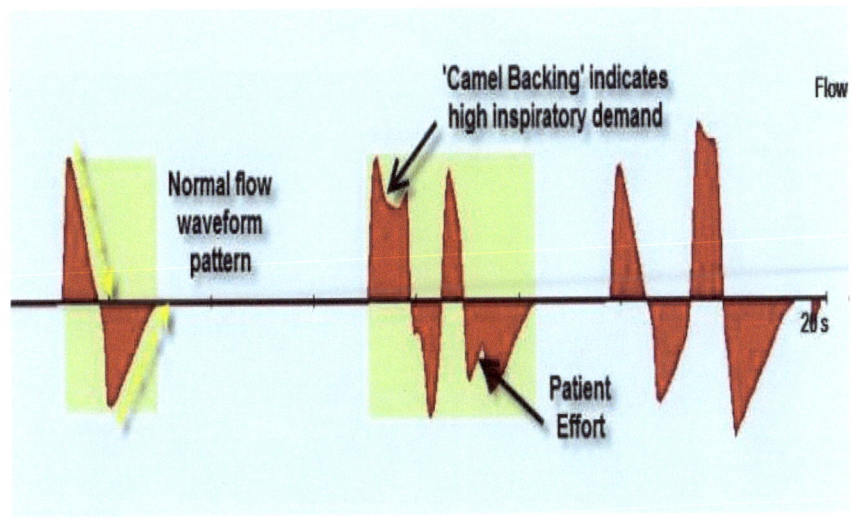

Image 45: Inadequate driving pressure as evidence by "camel backing" flow rising again.

Driving Pressure

Driving pressure or set pressure during ventilation in a pressure mode (PC-CMV, PC-IMV, PC-CSV) may also be inadequate for a patient's inspiratory demand. A peak pressure of 15-to-20 cmH2O is generally needed to provide significant support if the goal is to minimize patient work of breathing.

By observing the flow waveform the operator can identify an appropriate pressure setting to meet patients' demand. The flow waveform should have a constant linear deceleration to baseline then acceleration during the expiratory phase. Flow rising again during deceleration is evidence of an increased inspiratory drive and a peak pressure setting that is to low. This is termed "camel backing" because the flow waveform is shaped like a camels hump.

Driving Pressure

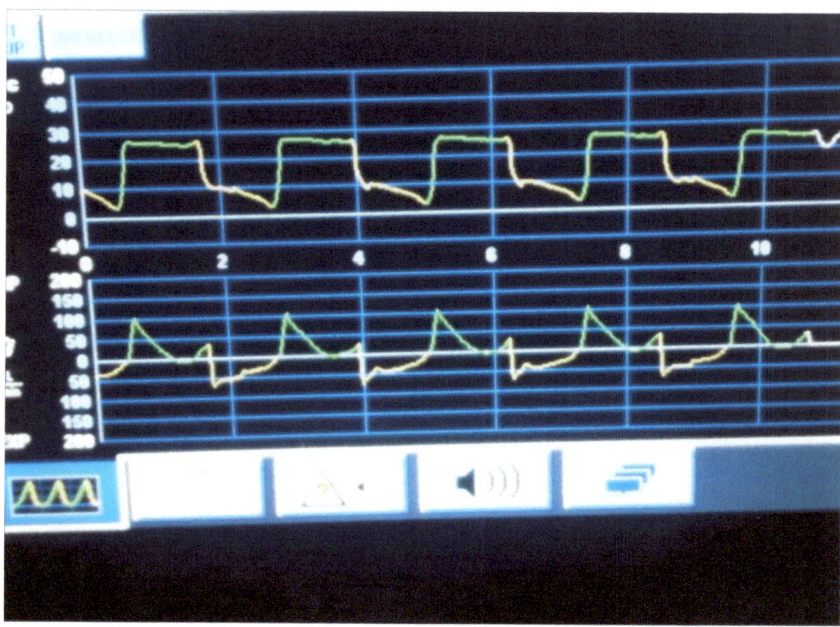

Image 46: Sepsis patient with a high inspiratory drive, even with the driving pressure set at 23 cmH2O, the patient is still flow hungry, as evidence from the flow rising again after deceleration.

If peak pressures are less than 30 cmH2O the operator may increase the pressure setting in 2 cmH2O increments until flow decelerates or up to 30 cmH2O peak inspiratory pressures (PIP).

Additionally, P0.1 can be evaluated to adjust driving pressure and/or the mode can be change to Proportional Assist Ventilation (PAV) or Neurally Adjusted Ventilatory Assist (NAVA), modalities that adjust pressure based on ventilatory drive.

Note- when increasing driving pressure the exhaled tidal volume may initially increase, but then decline as the ventilator off sets the patient's work of breathing. Also look for the P0.1 to decrease.

Caution- if increased ventilatory demand is a temporary event the patient is at a high risk for being over-assisted, which may lead to prolonged mechanical ventilation.

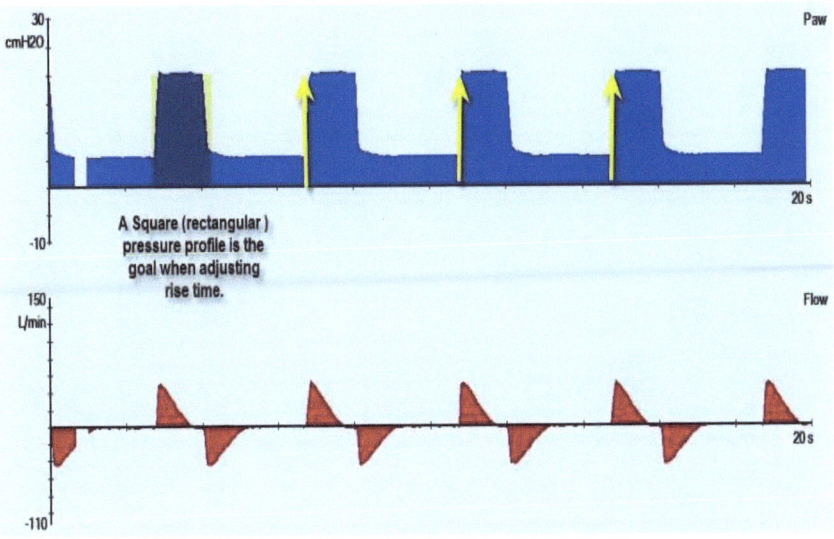

Image 47: Appropriate pressurization rate as evidence by the immediate rise in pressure after breath initiation creating a square pressure waveform.

Pressurization Rate

Also known as p-ramp, rise time, rise time percent, flow acceleration %, and slope, the pressurization rate is the time required for inspiratory pressure to rise to the set or target pressure. The pressurization rate setting allows the operator to fine tune the initial flow output during a pressure based breath (PC-CMV, PC-IMV, PC-CSV) to match the ventilator flow to the patients' inspiratory demand.

Inappropriate pressurization rates may result in elevated work of breathing, pressure over-shoot, premature termination of inspiration and/or prevention of the ventilator to attain the set inspiratory pressure.

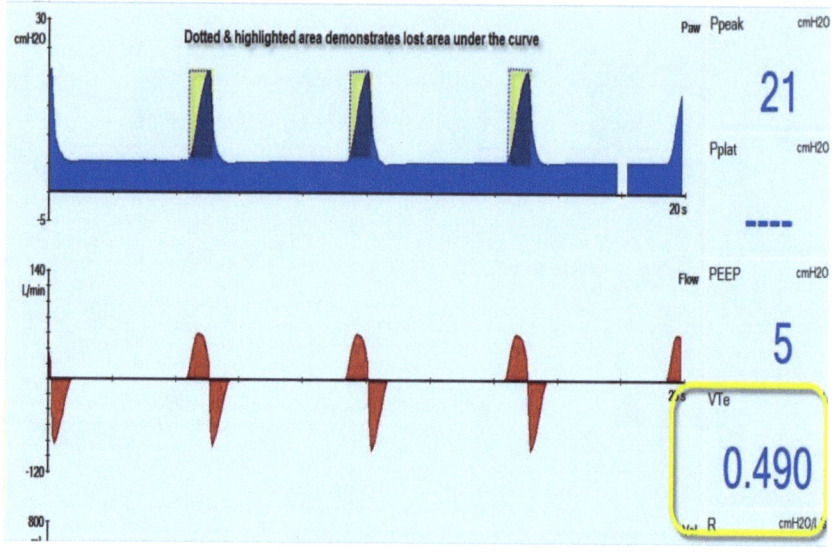

Image 48: Pressurization rate too slow, as evidence by the sloping pressure waveform.

Pressurization Rate that is Too Slow

A slow pressurization rate may cause increased work of breathing for patients with a high inspiratory drive and also decreases mean airway pressure, alveolar filling time, and area under the pressure curve (which may decrease delivered tidal volume).
In the above picture notice the measured tidal volume of 490, with a peak pressure of 21cmH2O. The following page demonstrates the increase in tidal volume (increased alveolar filling time) with the speeding up of the pressurization rate to achieve the optimal rectangular pressure waveform.
note- Tidal volume increases from 490 to 510 without increasing the set pressure, also notice that resistance and compliance remains the same.

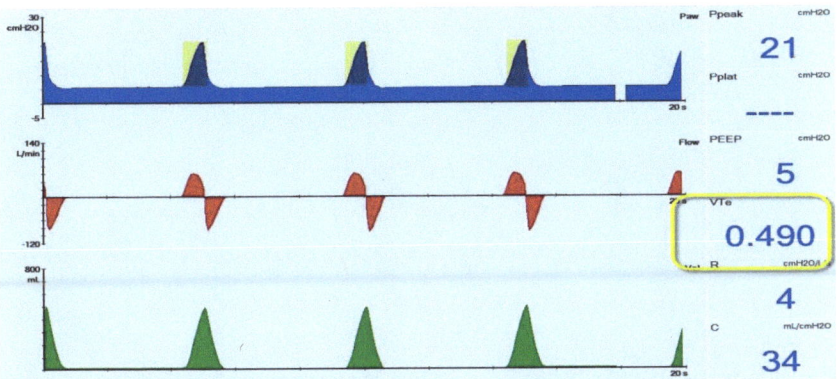

Image 49: Initial pressurization rate too slow notice the exhaled tidal volume of 490.

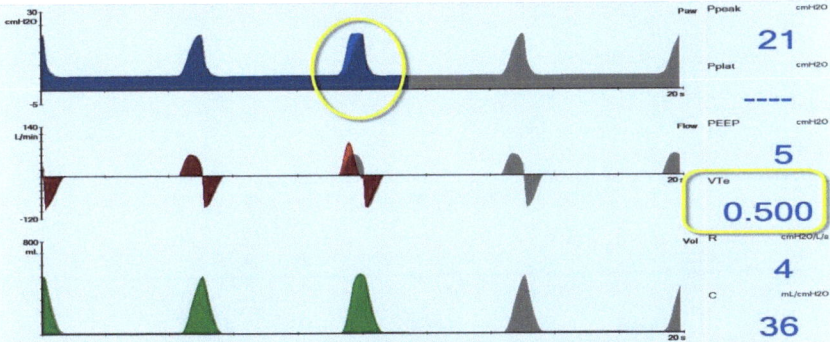

Image 50: Pressurization rate increased, notice the difference in shape (circled breath) tidal volume increased to 500.

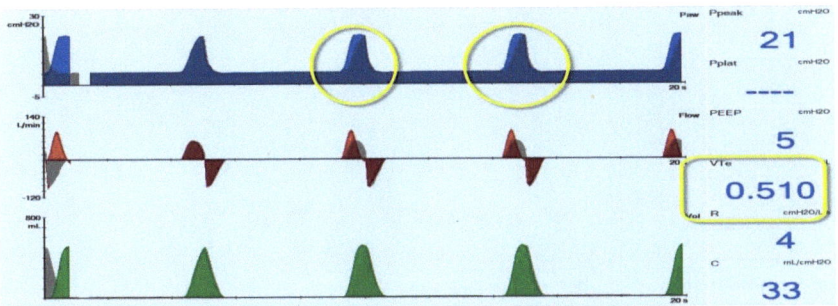

Image 51: Pressurization rate increased again, creating a larger tidal volume 510.

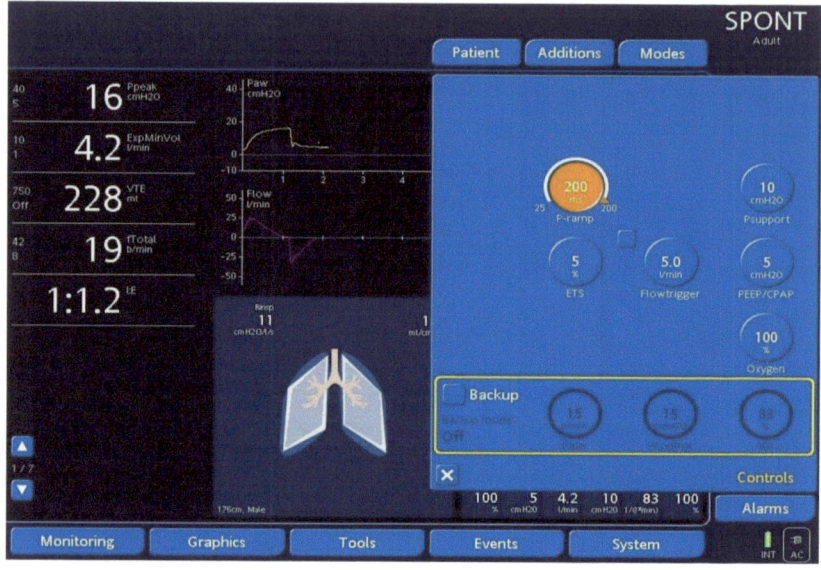

Image 52: Setting the pressurization rate to 200 milliseconds (0.2 Second) on the Hamilton G5 ventilator. This is an extremely long time for pressurization.

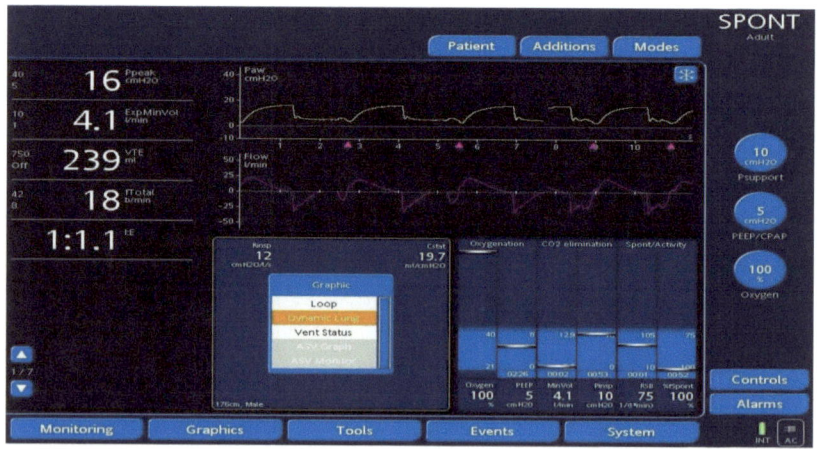

Image 53: Pressurization rate set at 0.2 second, notice the slow rise to peak pressure.

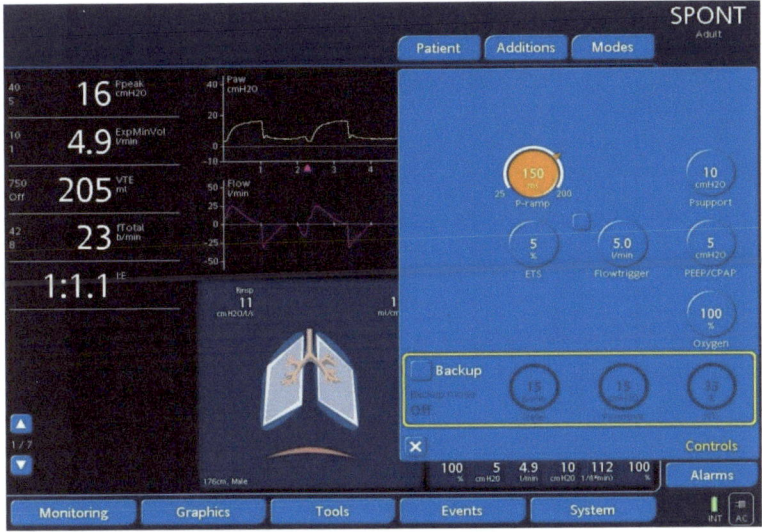

Image 54: Setting the pressurization rate to 0.15 second.

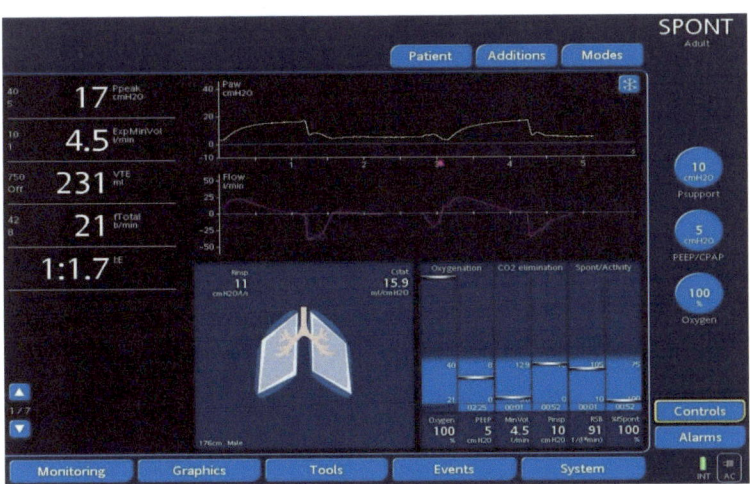

Image 55: Pressurization rate set to 0.15 seconds, still too slow.

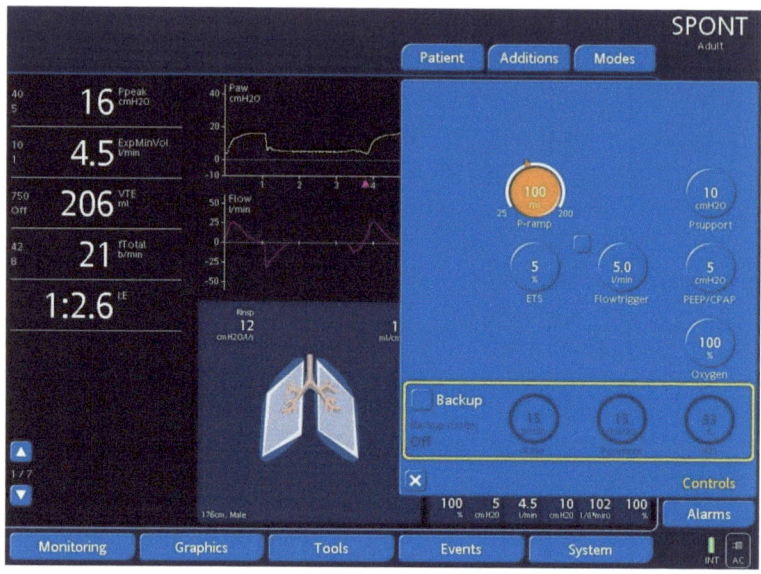

Image 56: Pressurization rate set to 0.1 second.

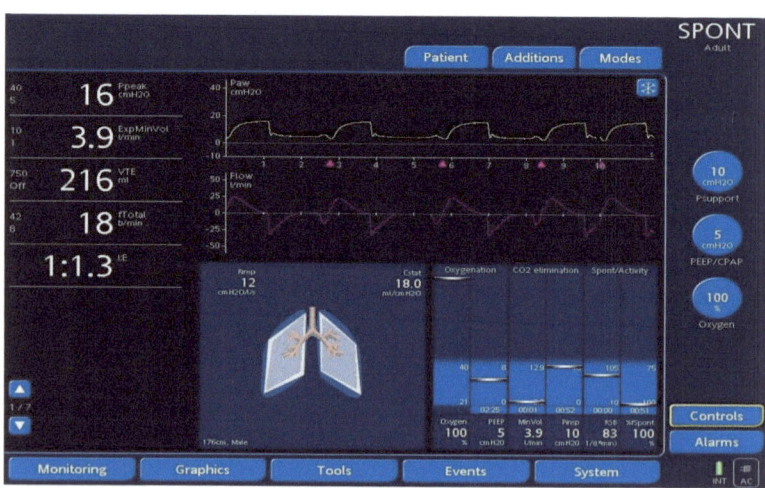

Image 57: Pressurization rate at 0.1 second, rate is still to slow however notice the pressure waveform is starting to square off.

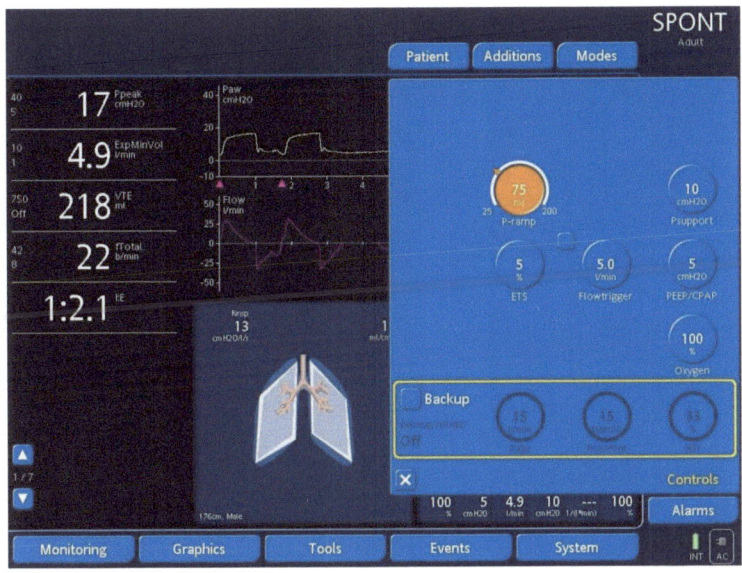

Image 58: Setting the pressurization rate to 0.075 Second.

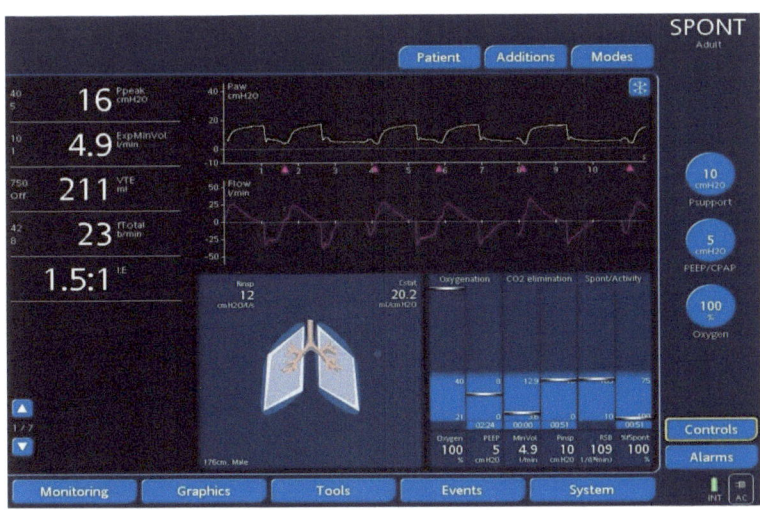

Image 59: Pressurization rate at 0.075 second.

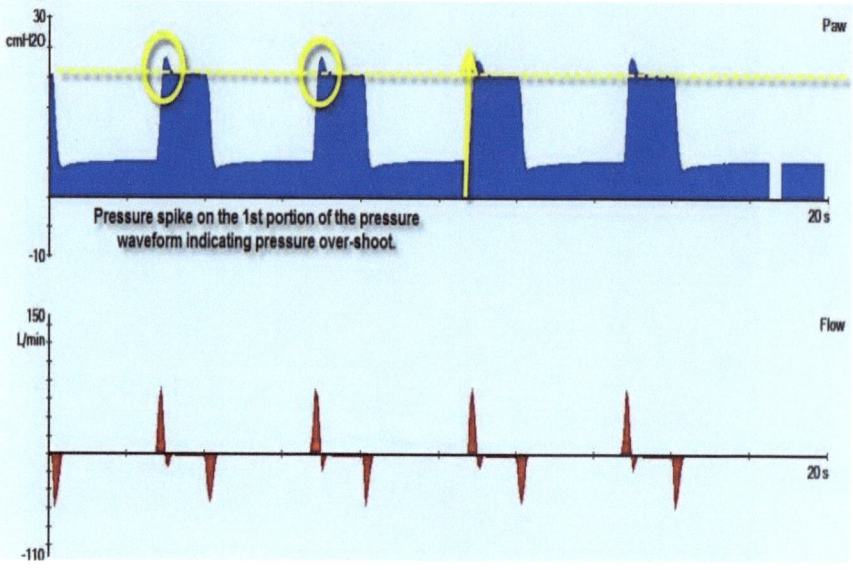

Image 60: Pressurization rate set too fast, as evidence by the pressure spikes going over the set pressure.

Pressurization Rate Too Fast

In lung models the fastest pressurization rates usually result in the lowest measured work of breathing, however increasing the pressurization rate above what is sufficient to meet the patients inspiratory demand does not provide further benefit in off loading work of breathing, and in fact may cause discomfort. Usually a moderate pressurization rate often results in the best patient ventilator synchrony [4, 12].

Setting the pressurization rate too fast especially in combination with a small E.T. tube or in patients with increased airway resistance may result in noticeable pressure over-shooting during the early stage of inspiration. This may lead to inappropriate termination of inspiration by setting off the pressure limitation threshold.

58

Pressurization Rate Too Fast

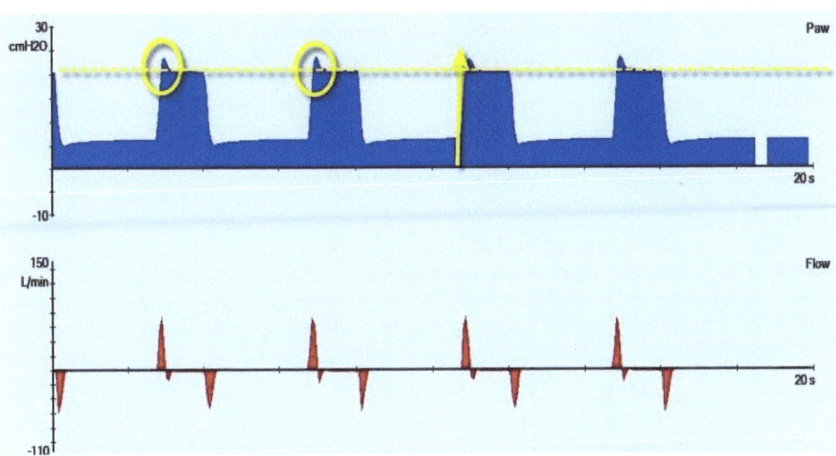

Image 61: Pressurization rate set too fast creating pressure spike over set inspiratory pressure.

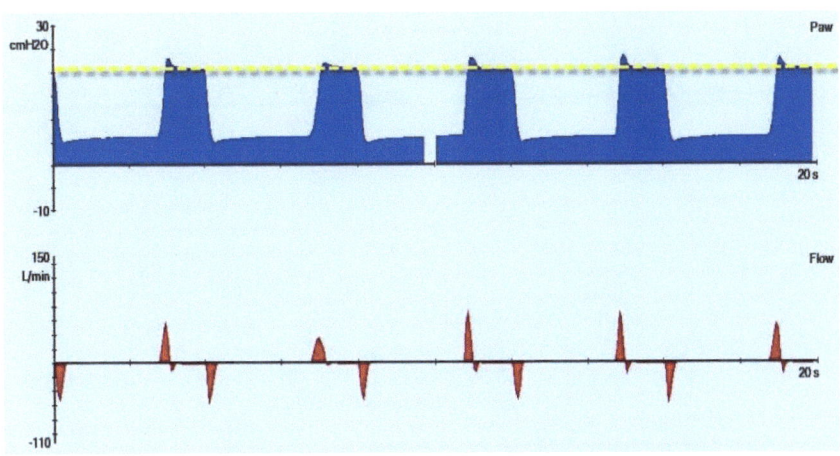

Image 62: Pressurization rate titrated to a slower rate however, it is still too fast.

Pressurization Rate Too Fast

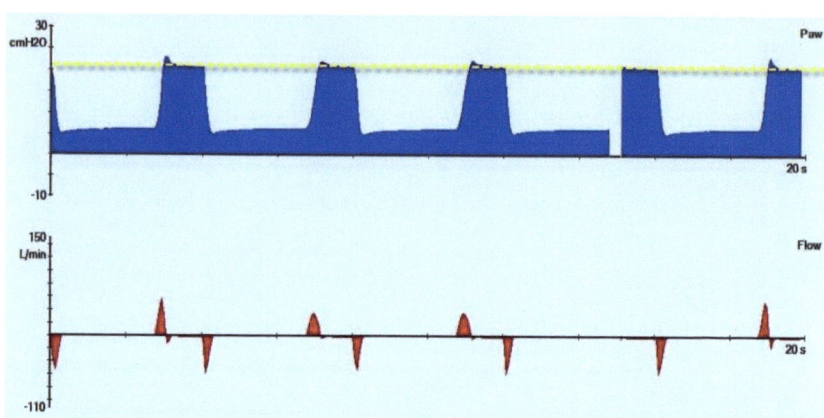

Image 63: Pressurization rate set slower, notice the pressure spike starting to decrease.

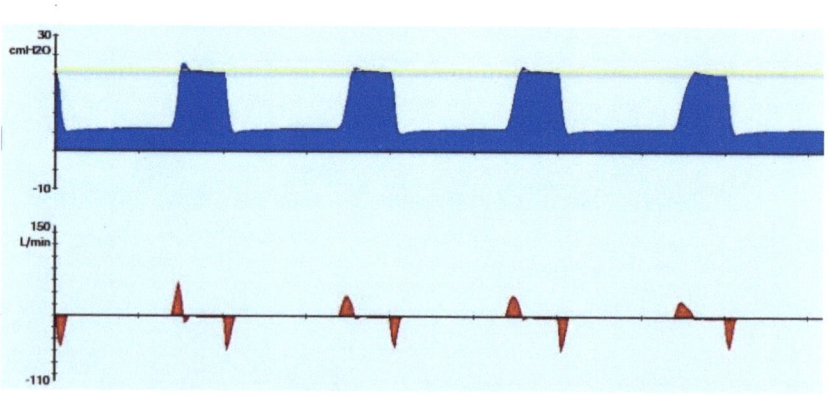

Image 64: Pressurization rate decreased to appropriate setting, notice the last breath the waveform is square without a pressure spike.

Flow Asynchronies

Conclusion

Flow asynchronies can be present in both volume based modalities and pressure based modalities. During volume ventilation (VC-CMV, VC-SIMV) flow mismatch can be a common asynchrony which is easily recognized and easily prevented. When utilizing pressure ventilation (PC-CMV. PC-IMV, PC-CSV) flow asynchronies are related to both a driving rate that is too low and inappropriate pressurization rate settings.

The operator can additionally consider using advance pressure based modes of ventilation (PAV, NAVA, ASV).
PAV & NAVA both modes provide unlimited inspiratory flow and decrease work of breathing by providing assistance proportional to the patients' demand (PAV) or relative assistance to the demand detected by a neural signal (NAVA).
ASV also provides unlimited inspiratory flow and prevents rapid shallow breathing by ensuring that the target tidal volume remains ≥ 4 ml/kg/IDBW.

Cycling Asynchronies

Premature Cycling
Delayed Cycling

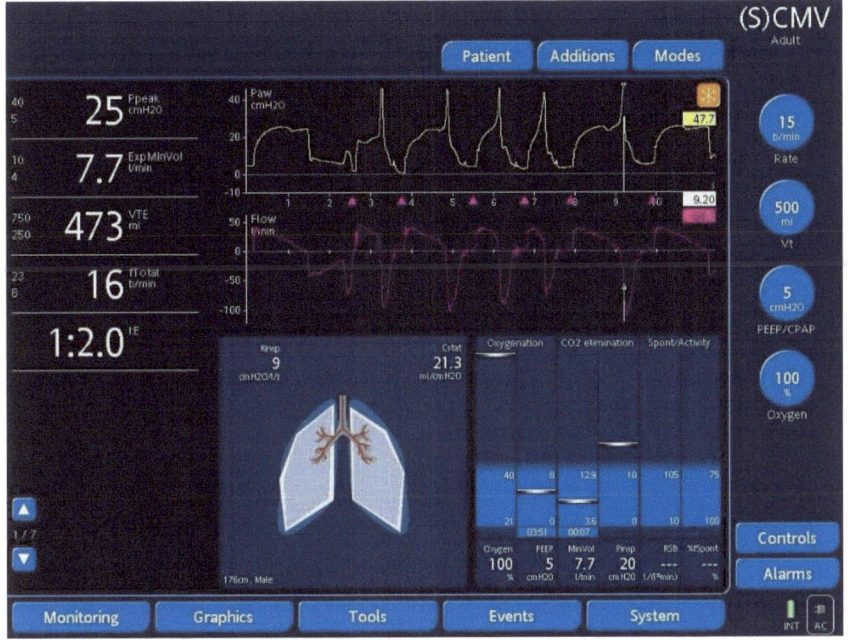

Image 65: Patient coughing, notice the peak pressure spikes (yellow pressure waveform) this may lead to premature cycling.

Premature Cycling

Premature cycling also known as premature termination or short cycling occurs when the ventilator breath cycle ceases abruptly, while the patient requires a longer inspiratory phase. It is defined by the delivered inspiratory time is less than 50% of the mean inspiratory time [1, 14].

Premature cycling may be attributed to pressure over-shots, causing the breath to cycle-off when the generated pressure meets the safety threshold setting. A good example of this is when a patient coughs during volume controlled ventilation (VC-CMV, VC-SIMV), in which the exhalation valve is closed throughout the set inspiratory time.

The following images (65-68) demonstrate premature cycling in a patient that is coughing.

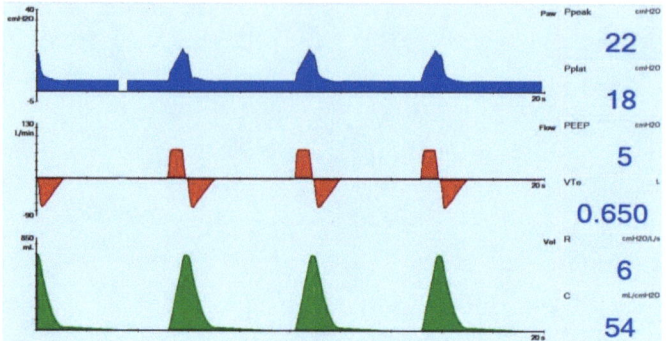

Image 66: Normal breath cycling during VC-CMV, the breath terminates with the set I-time.

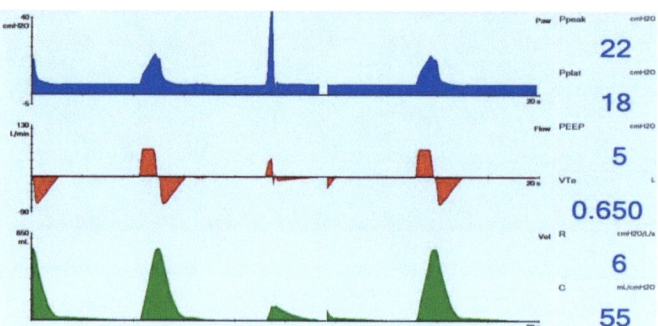

Image 67: One premature cycle present, notice the pressure spiking (blue pressure waveform) & short I-time.

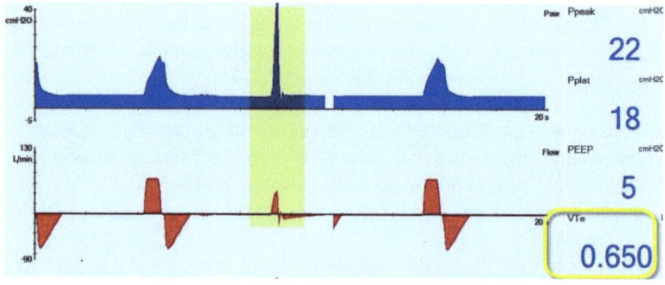

Image 68: Premature Cycle high-lighted in yellow notice this one event did not effect the exhaled tidal volume.

Premature Cycling

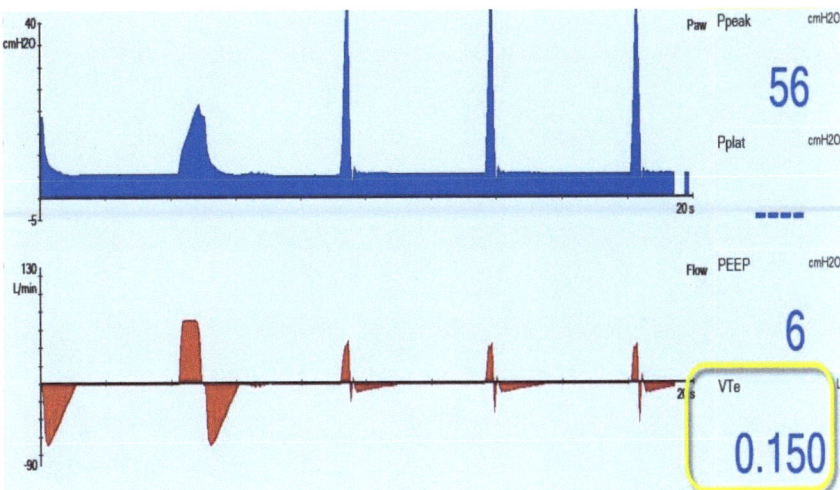

Image 69: A series of three premature cycles in a coughing patient, notice the drop in delivered tidal volume.

Premature cycling can be very uncomfortable to the patient and may lead to inadequate tidal volume delivery (as pictured above), too aggressive suctioning, over sedating the patient, and prolonged time on mechanical ventilation.

Premature Cycling

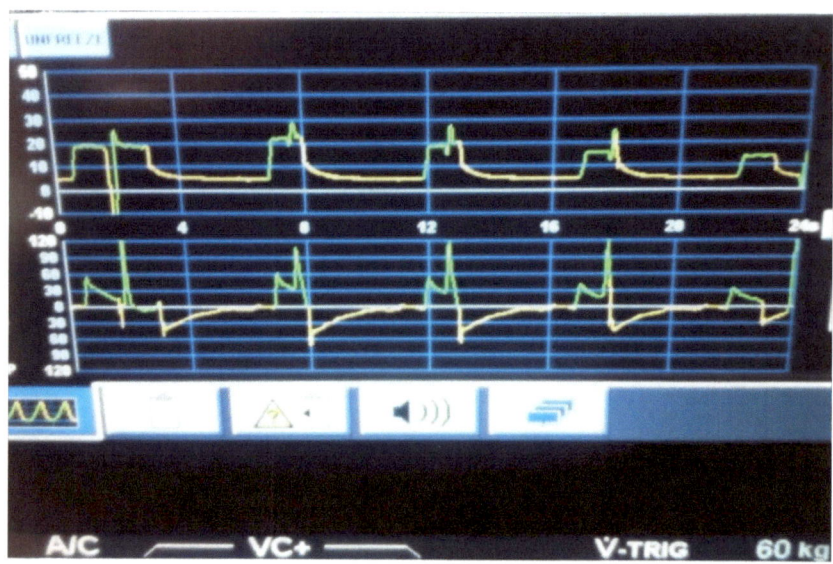

Image 70: Pressure and flow spikes caused by hiccups, which may lead to premature cycling.

Premature cycling can also happen during continuous spontaneous ventilation with pressure supported breaths. During CSV-PS the patient can more effectively end the breath based on their neural drive versus a set inspiratory time, however these spontaneous breaths still end based on a pre-set flow termination percentage.

During CSV-PS the operator may inappropriately set the pressurization rate too fast which leads to an initial pressure over-shoot. This over-shoot may exceed the set target pressure & terminate the inspiration prematurely as part of secondary breath termination criteria. The initial rapid rise in flow may also cause the breath to end earlier due to the pre-set flow termination point occurring sooner based on a higher initial peak inspiratory flow.

Premature Cycling

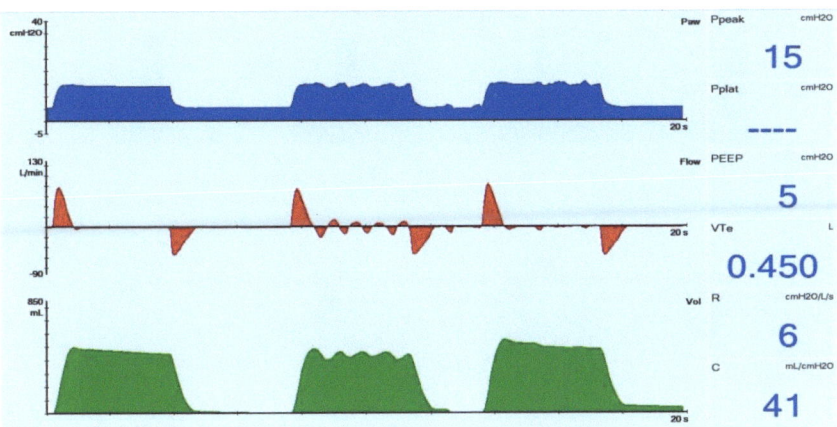

Image 71: Demonstrates the "floating" exhalation valve in action during the prolonged inspiratory phase (6 seconds) of Airway Pressure Release Ventilation.

One strategy to prevent premature cycling caused by pressure over-shooting is to utilize a pressure based mode of ventilation (e.g. PC-CMV, PC-SIMV, PC-CSV, or Adaptive Pressure Control). In newer generation ventilators the design of ventilator exhalation valves (e.g. active, floating) allows for unhindered spontaneous breathing during pressure based modalities.

The valve prevents the ventilator from terminating the inspiratory phase and losing mean airway pressure during coughing or exhalation.

Premature Cycling

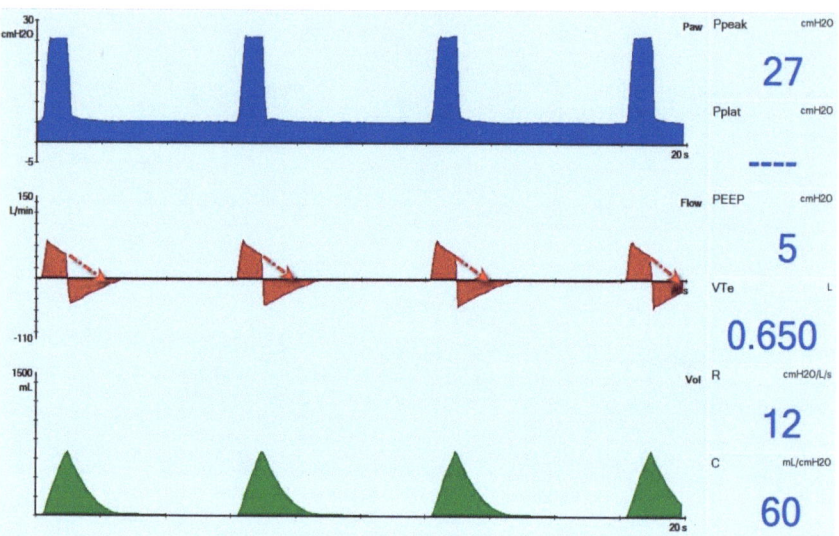

Image 72: I-time too short as evidence of the inspiratory flow waveform not fully decelerating to baseline (shown by the red arrow).

Premature cycling during breath delivery may be the result of an inspiratory time which is too short for the patient's inspiratory time constant, when utilizing PC-CMV or PC-IMV.

The above image demonstrates an I-time set too short as evidence of the inspiratory flow waveform not fully decelerating to baseline (shown by red the arrow).

Ideally the operator should titrate I-time to allow for full deceleration of the inspiratory flow waveform. When flow is allowed to fully decelerated, alveolar recruitment, alveolar ventilation, and mean airway pressure is maximized.

The following images (73-84) show the titrating of I-time to promote optimal V/Q matching.

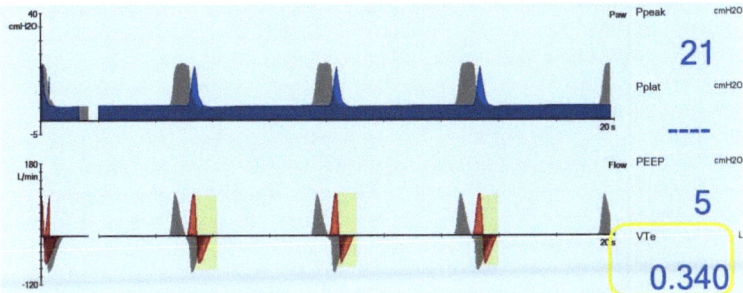

Image 73: Baseline I-time setting flow is not fully decelerating. Notice tidal volume of 340 ml.

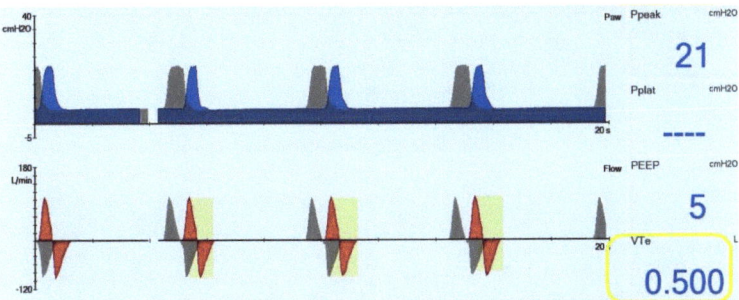

Image 74: I-time increased allowing for more lung recruitment tidal volume increases to 500 ml.

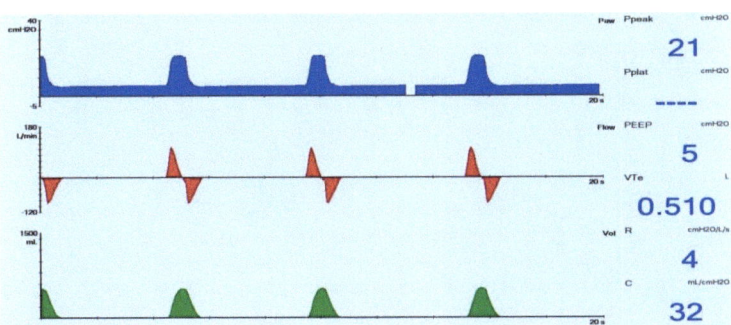

Image 75: I-time increased to allow for full deceleration of flow, tidal volume increases to 510ml.

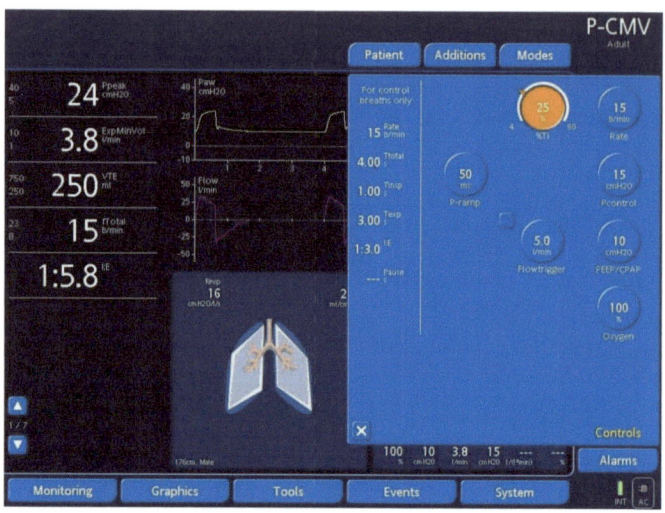

Image 76: Setting the I-time to 25%.

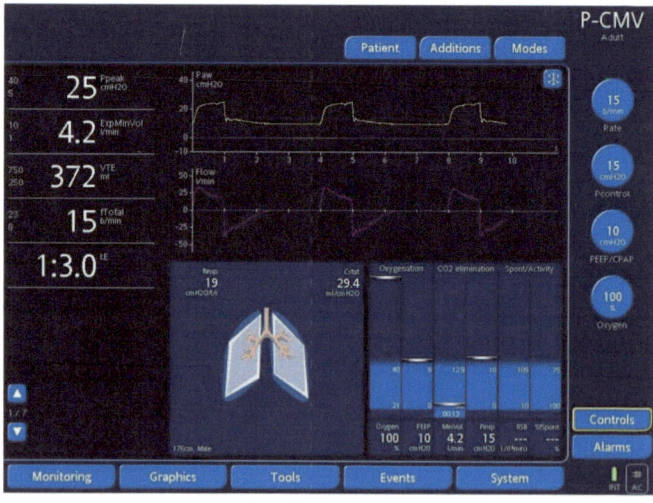

Image 77: I-time at 25% notice the flow waveform pattern (pink) & exhaled tidal volume of 372 ml.

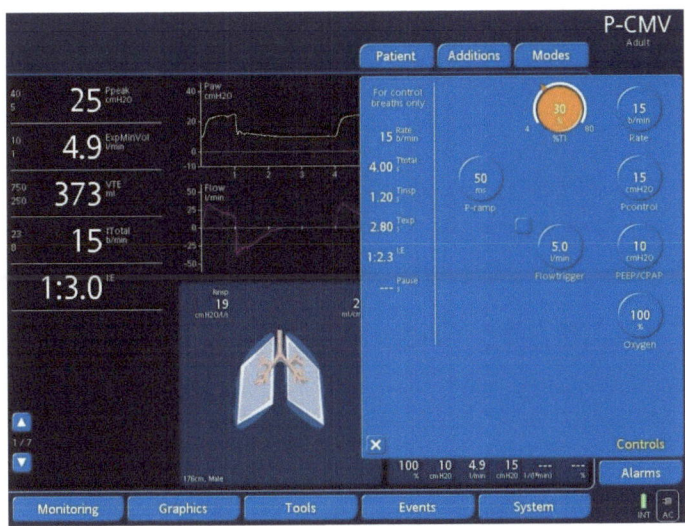

Image 78: I-time changed to 30%.

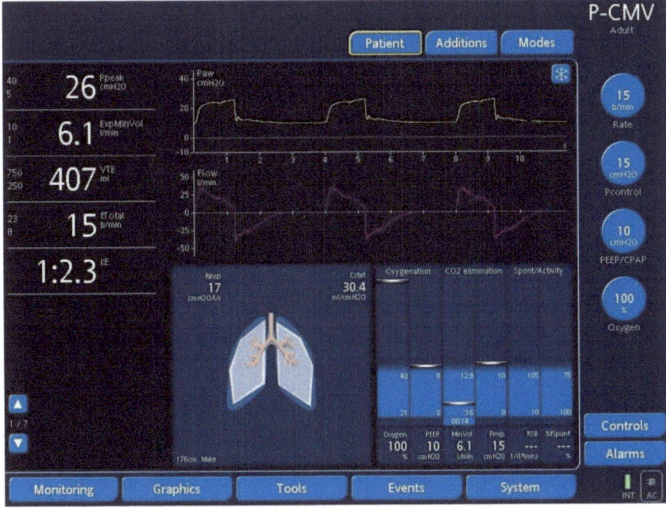

Image 79: I-time set at 30%, notice flow is allowed to decelerate further increasing the tidal volume from 373 to 407 ml.

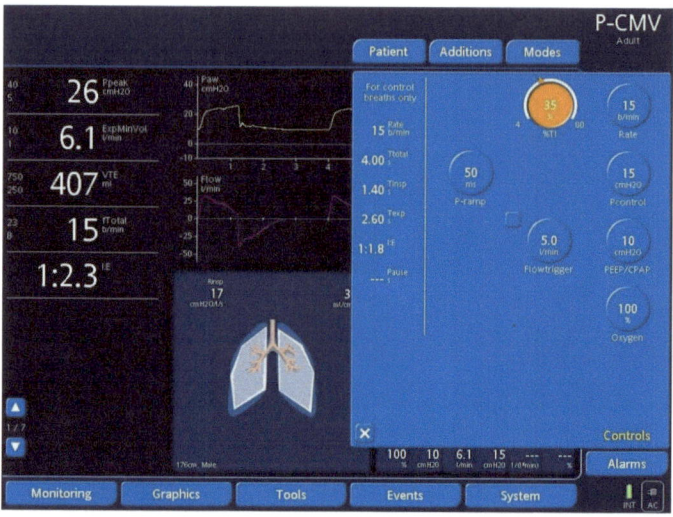

Image 80: Setting the I-time to 35%

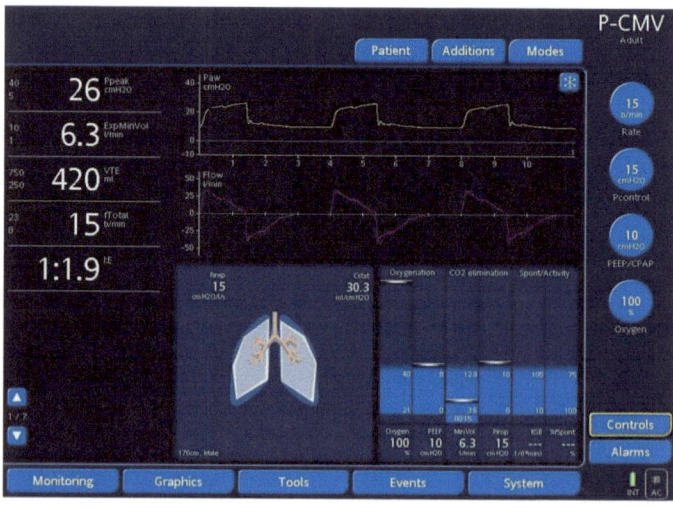

Image 81: I-time set at 35% flow is almost fully decelerating, tidal increases to 420ml.

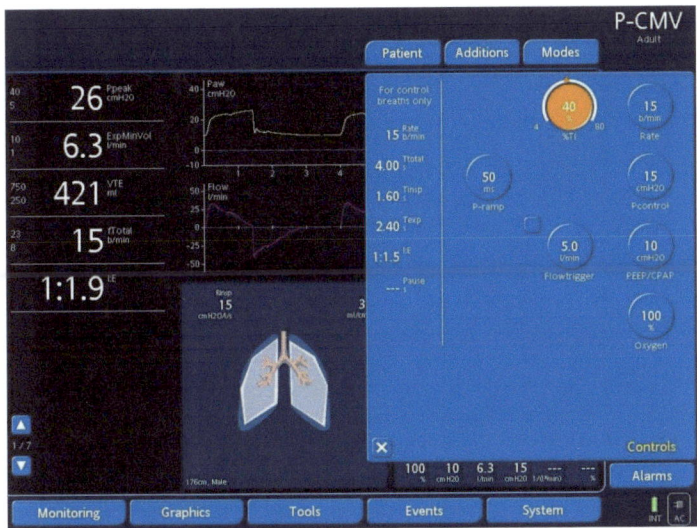

Image 82: I-time set at 40% increases tidal volume to 426ml shown in image 83).

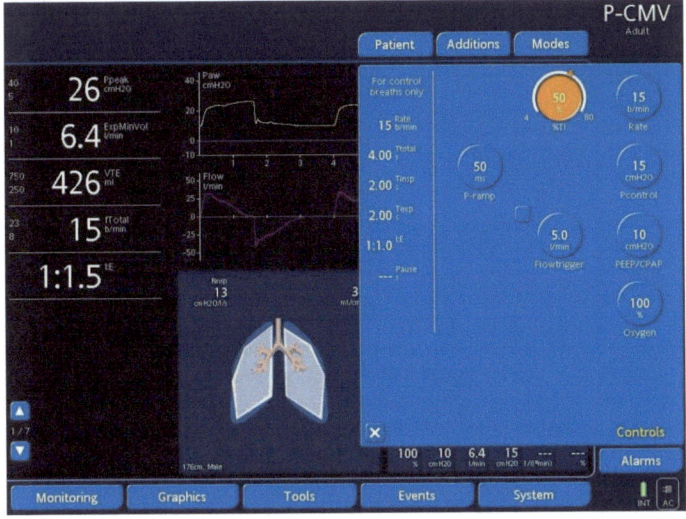

Image 83: I-time is set to 50%, notice baseline tidal volume of 426ml and flow was fully decelerating from the 40% I-time setting.

Premature Cycling

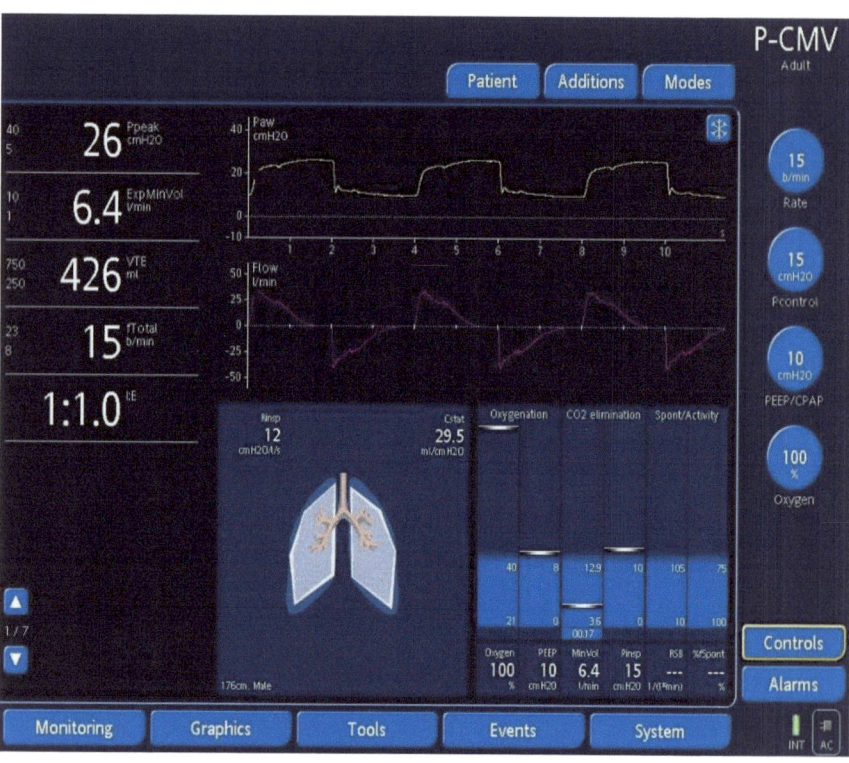

Image 84: I-time set at 50%, creates an inspiratory pause in this patient. Inspiratory pauses may increase mean airway pressure and prolong cycling.

Extending the I-time past the full deceleration point most likely will not increase the tidal volume. From the above image (84) one notices how the I-time was extended past the full deceleration point creating an inspiratory pause, this did not increase the tidal volume from the baseline of 426 ml which was generated from an I-time of 40% (image 83).

Creating an inspiratory pause will increase mean airway pressure and prolong the inspiratory phase which may cause discomfort and asynchrony in the patient. The ideal setting would end the ventilator inspiration corresponding with the end of the patient's neural inspiration.

Premature Cycling

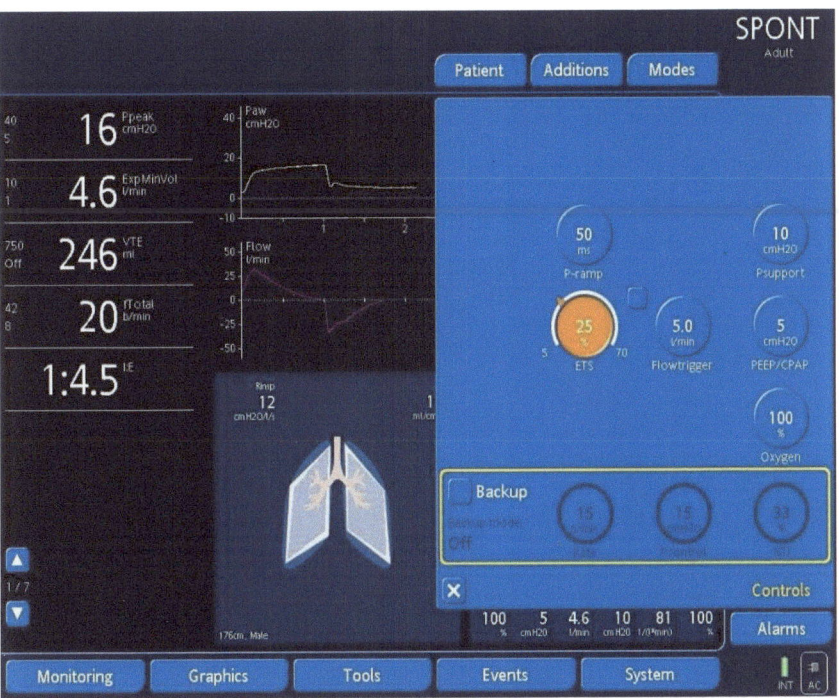

Image 85: The Expiratory Time Sensitivity setting (ETS) on a Hamilton G5 ventilator. This is the expiratory cycling threshold setting.

Expiratory Cycling Threshold

Premature cycling is also common during CSV-PS which additionally leads to double triggering, lower tidal volumes, higher respiratory rate & a higher work of breathing [14]. This is more prevalent in patients recovering from Acute Lung Injury (ALI).

Some newer generation ventilators allow for the adjustment of the expiratory cycling criteria providing the operator a way to improve matching between neural vs. machine cycling criteria.

Premature Cycling

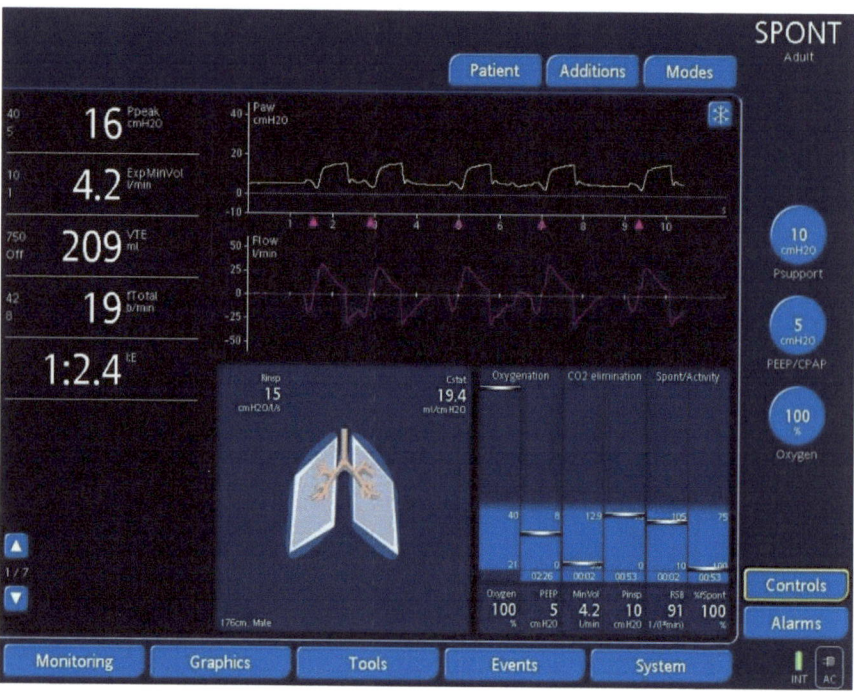

Image 86: ETS set at 25% notice the purple flow waveform & the amount of flow deceleration.

The expiratory cycling criteria during CSV-PS is based on a percentage of the peak inspiratory flow rate. From the previous image (85) the Expiratory Time Sensitivity (ETS) is set at 25%, which is a standard default, setting on most ventilators. This means that the breath will terminate when the flow decelerates to 25% above baseline. Another way to view this is to measure the peak inspiratory flow; the breath will terminated once 75% of the total peak expiratory flow is delivered.
Example: peak inspiratory flow 100 liters/second, the breath will terminate when the flow decelerates to 25 liters/second.

Note- on most ventilators a smaller ETS setting equals a longer breath.

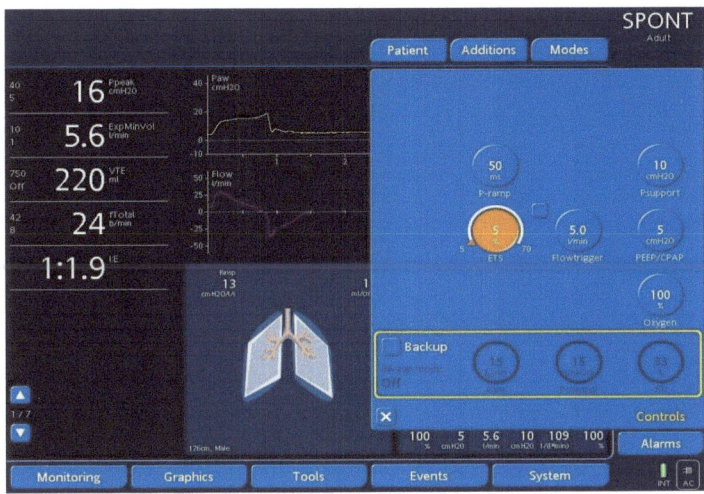

Image 87: In patients recovering from ALI the operator may need to increase the expiratory cycle criteria to provide optimal patient comfort. Notice the ETS setting of 5%.

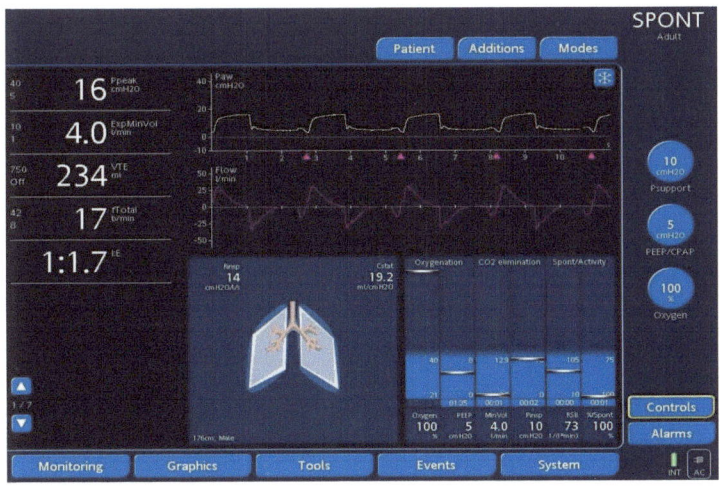

Image 88: ETS set at 5% notice that flow almost fully decelerates, allowing for a larger tidal volume.

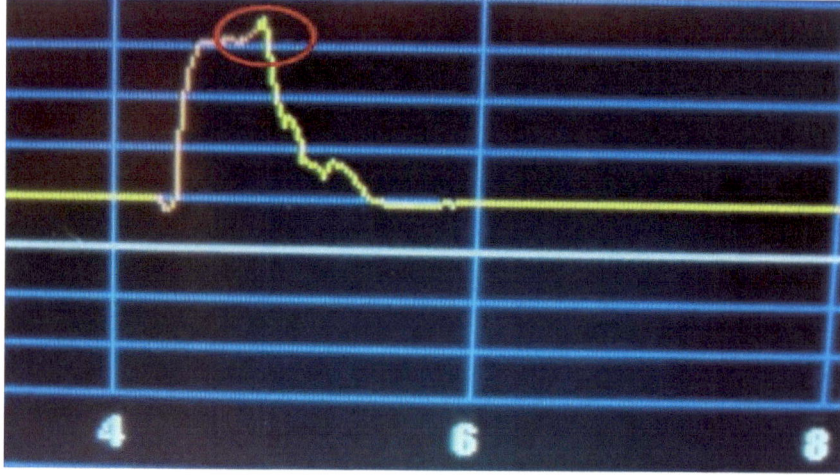

Image 89: Pressure spike at the end of inspiration may indicate the presence of active expiratory effort before the cycle criteria is met.

Delayed Cycling

Delayed cycling also known as prolonged cycling or prolonged termination is described as "when the ventilator breath cycle is longer than the patient inspiratory time (mechanical I-time is > neural I-time)" [4]. It also has been quantified as the I-time is twice as long as the mean I-time [1].

Basically delayed cycling is "the presence of active expiratory effort before the cycle criteria is met" [14].

One form of delayed cycling has been previously mentioned, that is when the operator inappropriately sets the inspiratory time too long. However, delayed cycling is also very common during CSV-PS.

A pressure spike at the end of inspiration as pictured (image 89) may indicate delayed cycling however this is not always associated with expiratory muscle activity. The spike may also be due to the relaxation of the inspiratory muscles, the spike is caused by the returning of pressure creating a temporary increase in pressure (usually associated with higher levels of pressure support > 10 cmH2O).

Always evaluate the patient for distress to determine if it is delayed cycling vs. muscle relaxation. If the patient looks relaxed and the P0.1 is within limits then the spike is most likely due to muscle relaxation.

Delayed Cycling

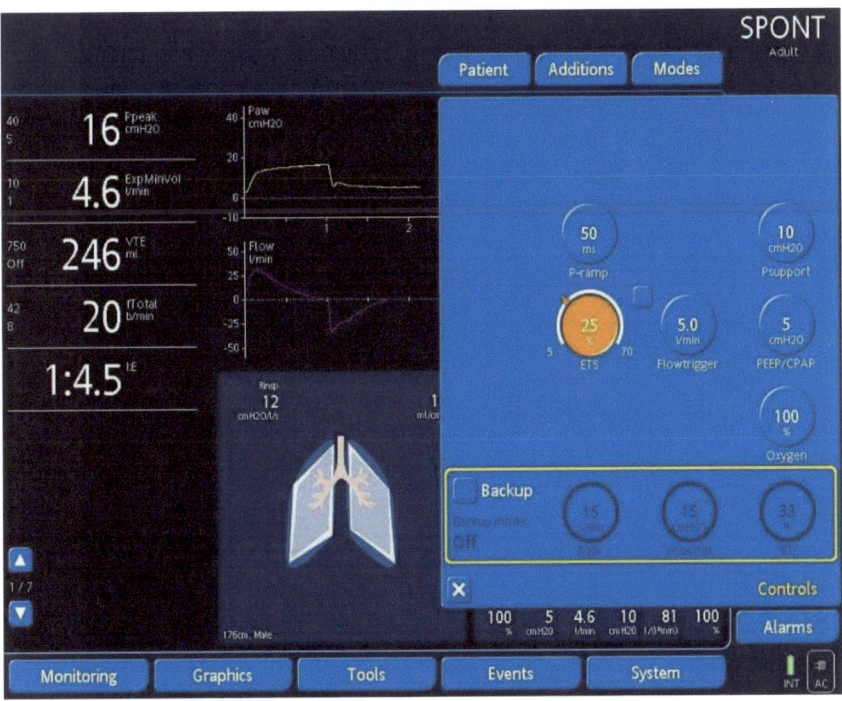

Image 90: ETS setting at 25% a standard default setting on most ventilators.

A 25% expiratory cycling threshold is a common default setting in most mechanical ventilators. This setting is appropriate in a large percent of the patient population. As previously mentioned a default setting of 25% may be too short in patients recovering from ALI, conversely, in patients with histories of airway obstruction this setting may be too long.

Prolonged expiratory cycling in the COPD patient may increase work of breathing, intrinsic PEEP, and trigger asynchronies (ineffective efforts) [14].

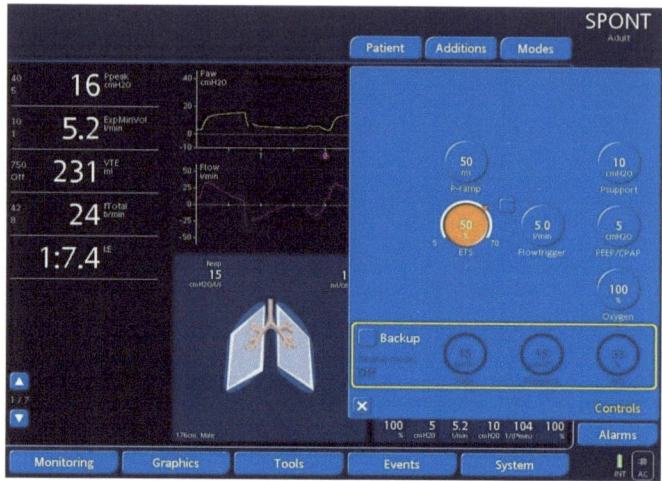

Image 91: For COPD patients changing the ETS to cycle the breath earlier decreases ineffective efforts and improves patient ventilator synchrony. ETS changed to 50%.

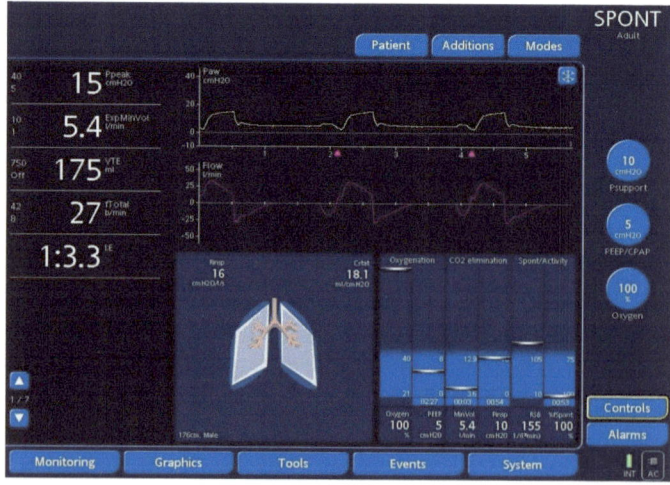

Image 92: ETS set at 50% notice the flow (purple) waveform and how the breath ends sooner, based on the percentage of flow deceleration.

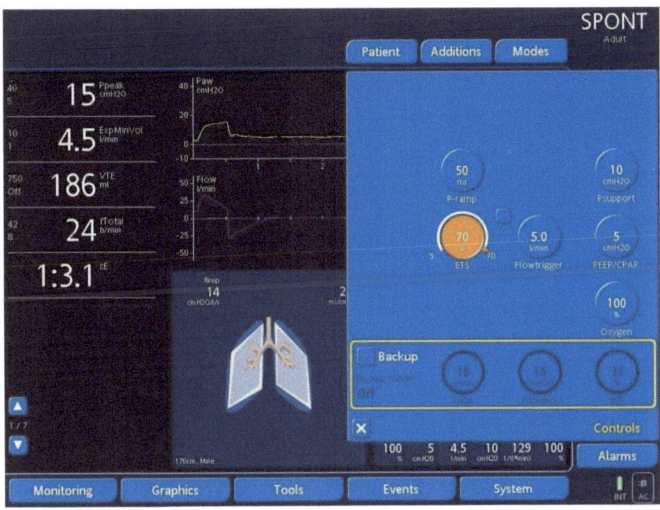

Image 93: One way to titrate ETS is to change the setting by 5% until ineffective efforts disappear. ETS setting changed to 70%.

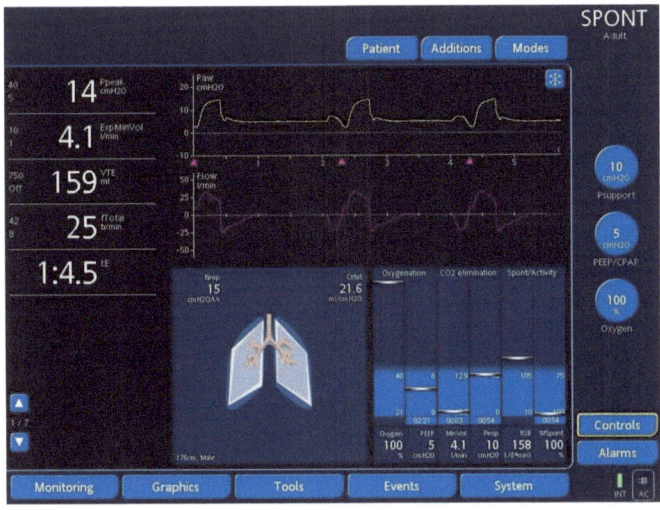

Image 94: ETS setting at 70% the breath terminates at 30% of the peak inspiratory flow. Notice how much shorter the breath is.

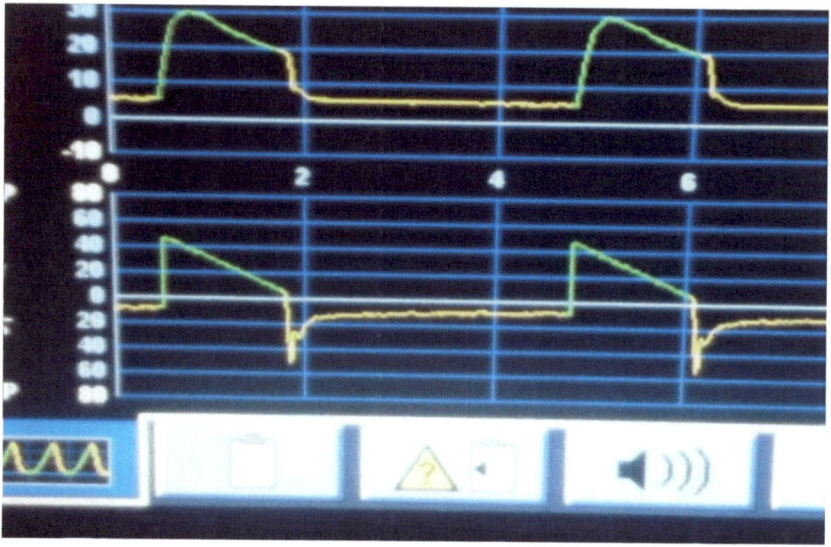

Image 95: Prolonged expiratory emptying, notice the prolonged expiratory phase (bottom flow waveform) lasting longer than 3 seconds.

Expiratory Asynchrony

Expiratory asynchrony is the "delay in the relaxation of the expiratory muscle activity prior to the next mechanical inspiration" [14]. Delayed expiratory emptying increases PEEPi.

PEEPi is the difference between the total PEEP and the external PEEP thus provides information on the amount of dynamic hyper-inflation working on the respiratory system and on all the intra-thoracic organs. PEEPi has the same adverse effects of PEEP concerning both hemodynamics, barotrauma, and volutrauma.

PEEPi affects patient triggering by creating a load that the patient has to overcome. PEEPi is easily quantified by utilizing an end-expiratory occlusion maneuver (automated on most newer ventilators).

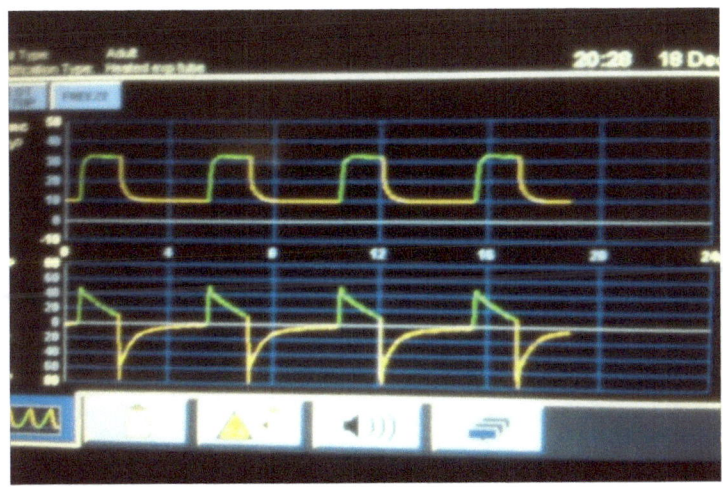

Image 96: Evaluating the expiratory flow waveform, one would assume there is no PEEPi present. Conversely, this should be quantified by using an end-expiratory occlusion maneuver.

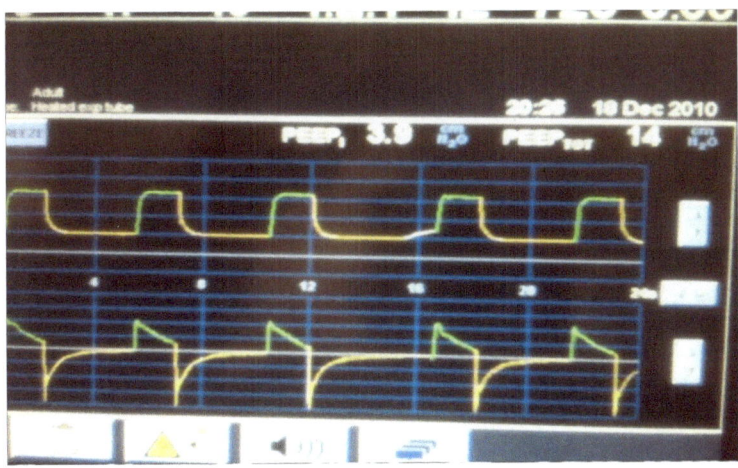

Image 97: Same patient as in image 96, after an end-expiratory maneuver. Notice a total PEEP of 14 cmH2O & a PEEPi of 3.9 cmH2O. There should be no PEEPi, a moderate amount is 2-to-6 cmH2O, & a high amount is > 8 cmH2O.

Expiratory Asynchrony

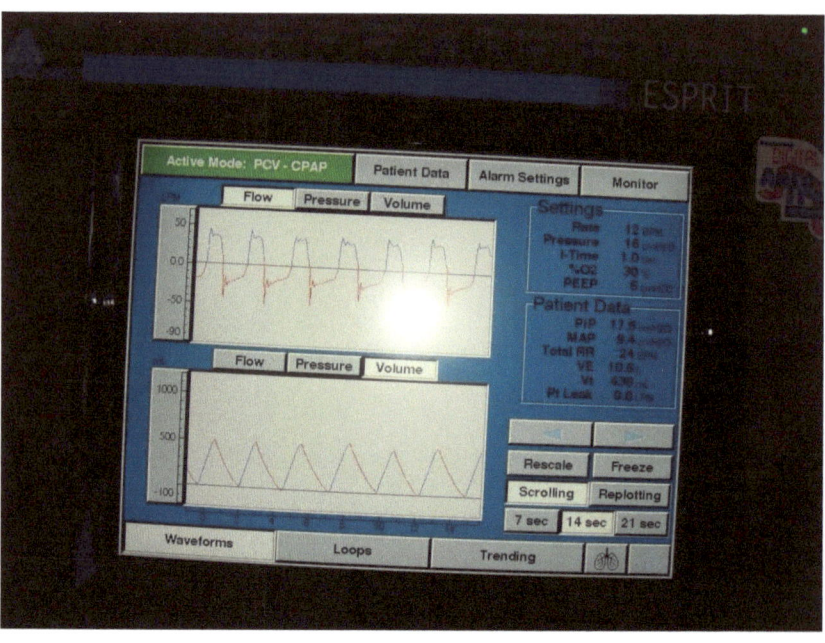

Image 98: The top waveform (flow) shows airway obstruction by evidence of the expiratory flow not returning to baseline.

Intrinsic PEEP can occur in the absence of expiratory flow limitation, under conditions of high minute ventilation, and/or increased equipment resistance (e.g. mucus narrowed E.T. tube, clogged Heat Moisture Exchangers, or expiratory filters).

The above image (98) provides an example of PEEPi caused by a Heat Moisture Exchanger (HME) placed in-line with the ventilator circuit. HME's and filters on the expiratory limb can become clogged creating additional expiratory resistance and PEEPi.

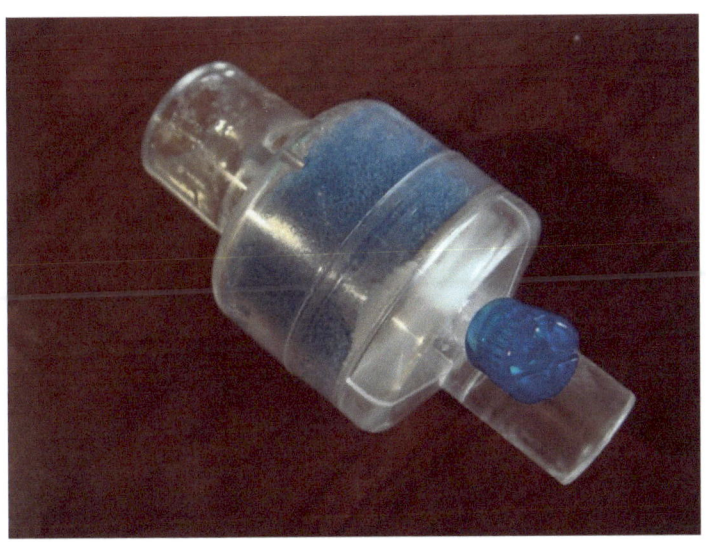

Image 99: Clogged HME from patient example image 98.

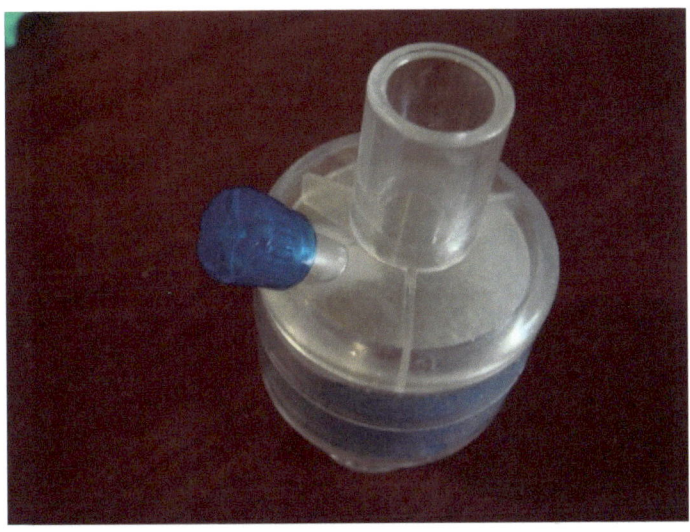

Image 100: Clogged HME secondary to secretions, patient example image 98.

Expiratory Asynchrony

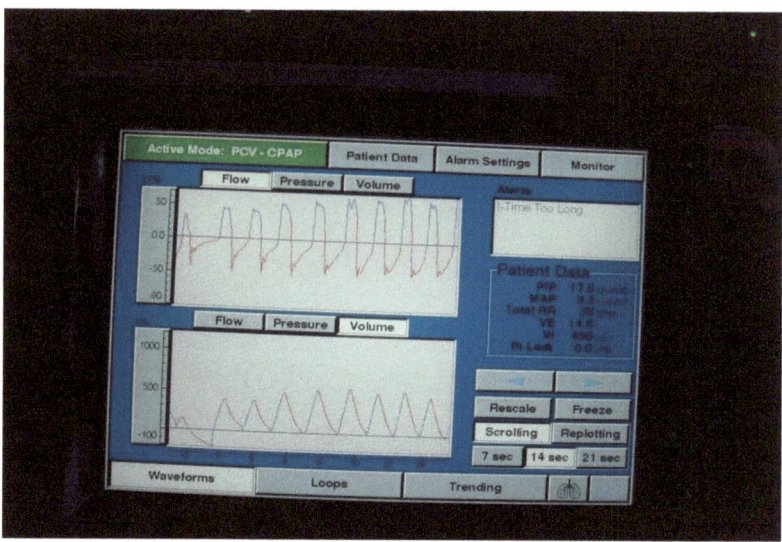

Image 101: Same patient as image 98 after HME replaced, notice changing the HME eliminated the expiratory obstruction.

To decrease expiratory asynchrony always evaluate the patient's airway first for obstructions or secretions. Assess lung sounds for wheezes, the patient may need bronchodilators. To decrease PEEPi reduce the minute ventilation and lengthen the expiratory time.

To reduce the triggering load from the PEEPi apply a small amount of circuit PEEP. Increase the PEEP by 2 cmH2O until there is no longer a trigger delay, or a reduction in ineffective efforts. The patient should also appear more comfortable.

Once you synchronize expiratory asynchrony you automatically eliminate all ineffective efforts (see images 36-38) and you get one-to-one relationships between the patient rate and the measured respiratory rate.

Expiratory Asynchrony

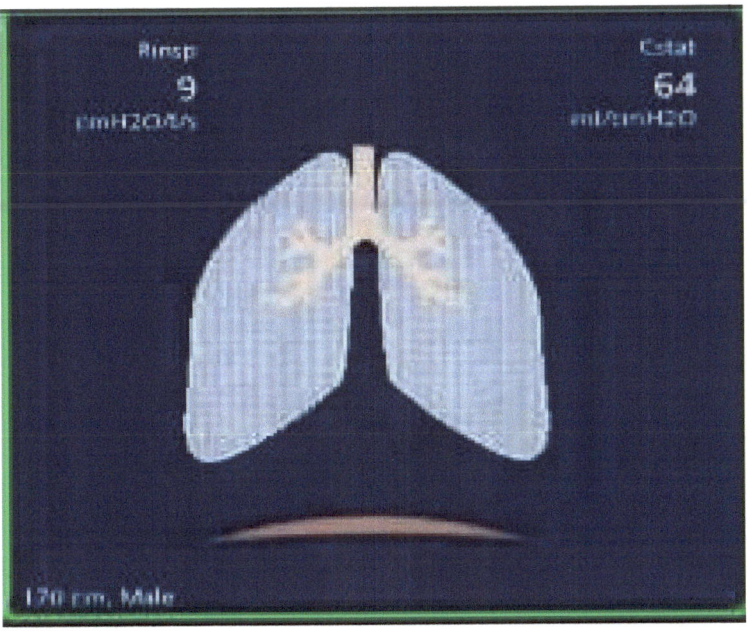

Image 102: The "Dynamic Lung" on a Hamilton G5 ventilator showing normal pulmonary mechanics.

Other ways to identify expiratory asynchrony or expiratory flow obstruction include evaluating the expiratory time constant (RCexp) and observing the "Dynamic Lung"® (™ Hamilton Medical, Reno, NV).

The RCexp calculates the rate at which the lungs empty. In adults an RCexp > 1.2 seconds indicates airway obstruction.

Expiratory Asynchrony

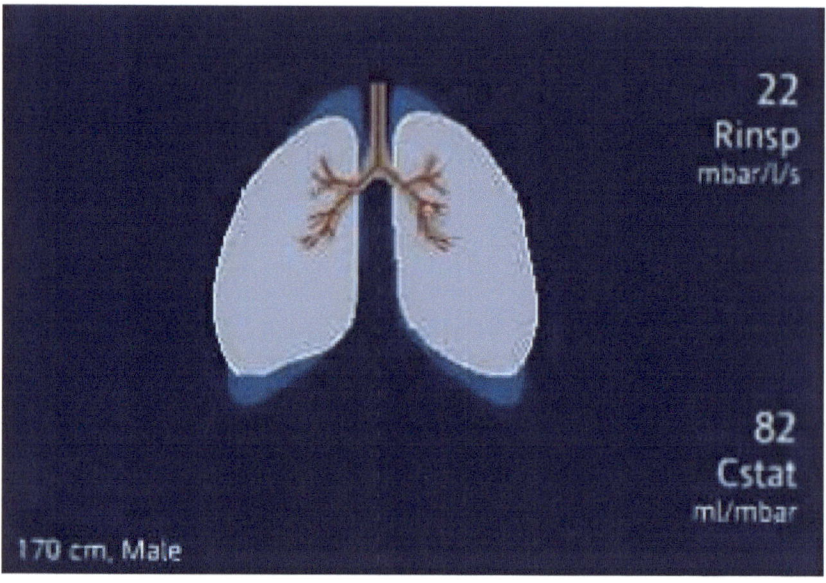

Image 103: The "Dynamic Lung" showing Airway obstruction, notice the measured resistance of 22 & the red narrowed bronchial tree.

The Dynamic Lung is an innovative tool that provides the operator with a visual representation of the patient's pulmonary mechanics. The tool changes its shape and colors based on changes in the respiratory system. It is very useful since the operator does not need to scroll through multiple screens reviewing data associated with lung mechanics.

VENTILATOR	ADAPTIVE CONTROL MODE
Draeger	AutoFlow
Hamilton Medical	Adaptive Pressure Ventilation
Maquette Servo-i	Pressure Regulated Volume Control Volume Support
Puritan Bennett 840	Volume Control +
Newport E500	Volume Target Pressure Control
Viasys	Pressure Regulated Volume Control

Image 104: Commercial names for ventilator modes the use Adaptive Pressure Control.

Adaptive Pressure Control

Adaptive pressure control (APC) modalities have specific asynchronies in relation to the inspiratory flow phase of breath delivery.

During APC the pressure limit of the ventilator is automatically adjusted over several breaths to maintain a target tidal volume (set by the operator) as the patient's condition changes.

The ventilator compares the measured exhaled tidal volume with the target tidal volume to determine if the driving pressure is increased (delivered Vt < target Vt), or remain constant or decreased (delivered Vt > or = target tidal volume).

The following images (105-108) demonstrate the titration of the driving pressure to maintain a target tidal volume, during increases in lung compliance.

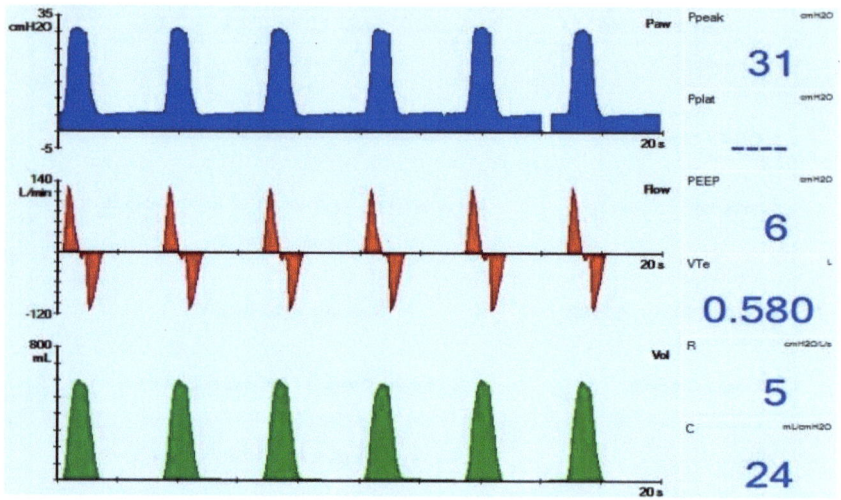

Image 105: Baseline Screen shot of APC with a target Vt of 600 ml, Resistance of 5 & Compliance of 24, PIP 31 cmH20.

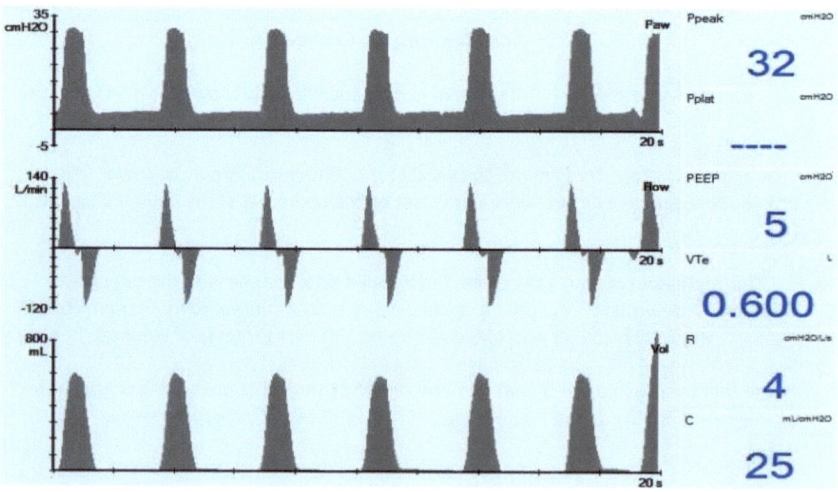

Image 106: Baseline Screen shot of APC with waveforms changed to grey to show progressive changes.

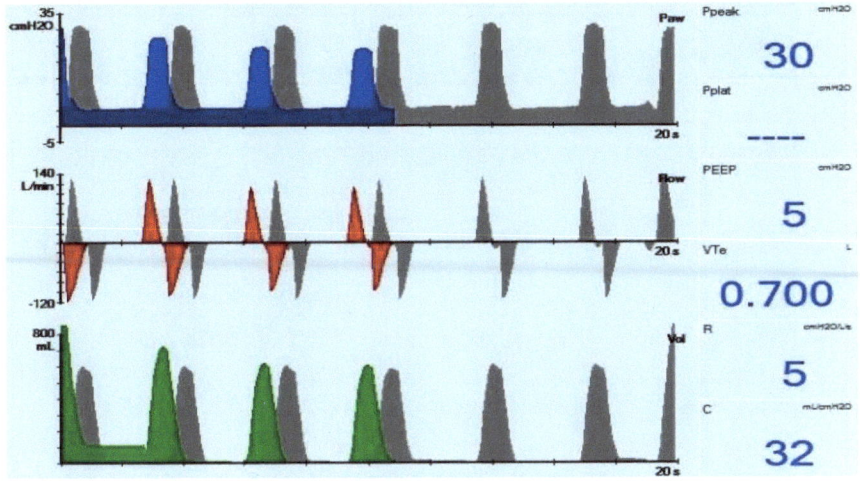

Image 107: APC after increase in compliance (32) measured Vt at 700 ml so pressure starts to titrate down.

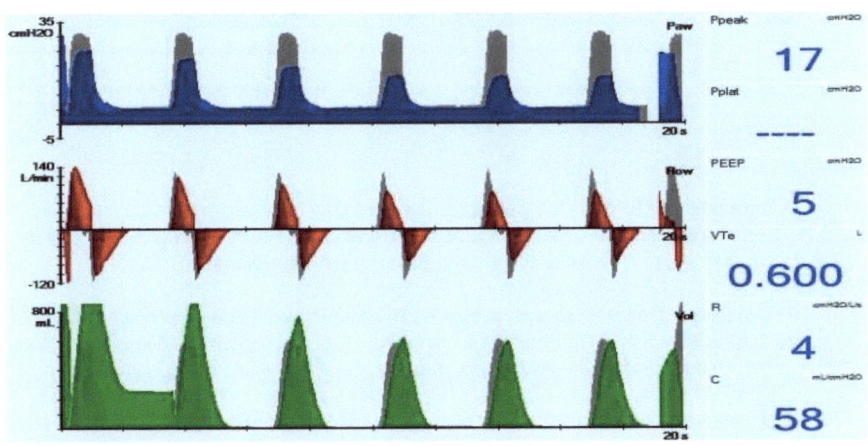

Image 108: APC pressure continues to titrate down (to 17 cmH2O) to obtain a target Vt of 600 ml after compliance increases to 58.

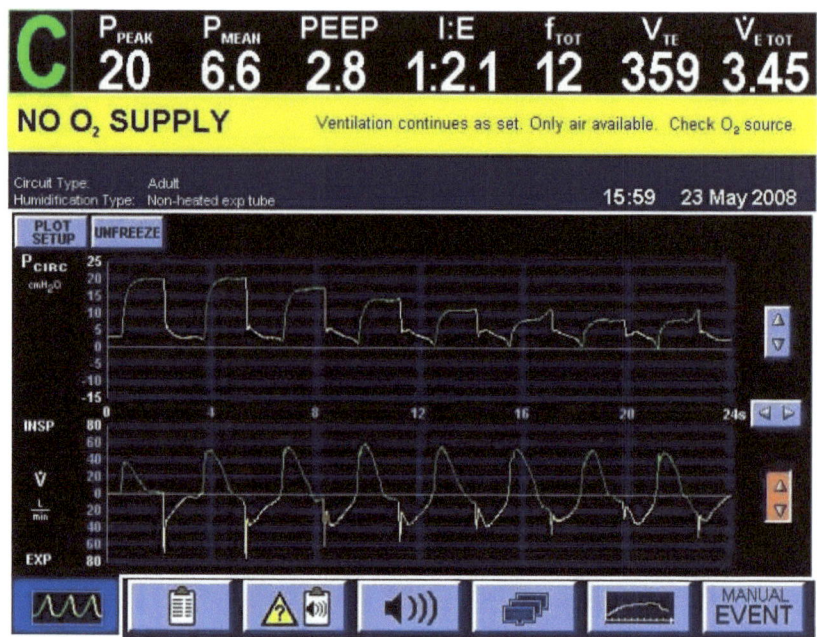

Image 109: APC premature decrease in driving pressure (PIP started at 20 cmH20 & decreased to ~ 9 cmH20) secondary to increased inspiratory effort.

Since pressure titration is based upon delivered tidal volume the pressure limit may prematurely decrease in patients with an increased inspiratory effort generating tidal volumes far greater than the set tidal volume.

This inadequate peak inspiratory pressure can become a common occurrence if utilizing APC in patients with a high metabolic demand (e.g. burns, sepsis), head injury, or ARDS patients ventilated with a low tidal volume strategy (4-6 ml/kg/IDBW).

Since APC modalities are fundamentally pressure control modes (in regards to basic breath delivery), all aspects of pressure ventilation must be considered (I-time, Pressurization rate). As previously mentioned; a peak pressure of 15-to-20 cmH2O is needed to
relieve work of breathing in the critically ill patient.
Consider evaluating the P0.1 to help determine comfort level.

Adaptive Pressure Control

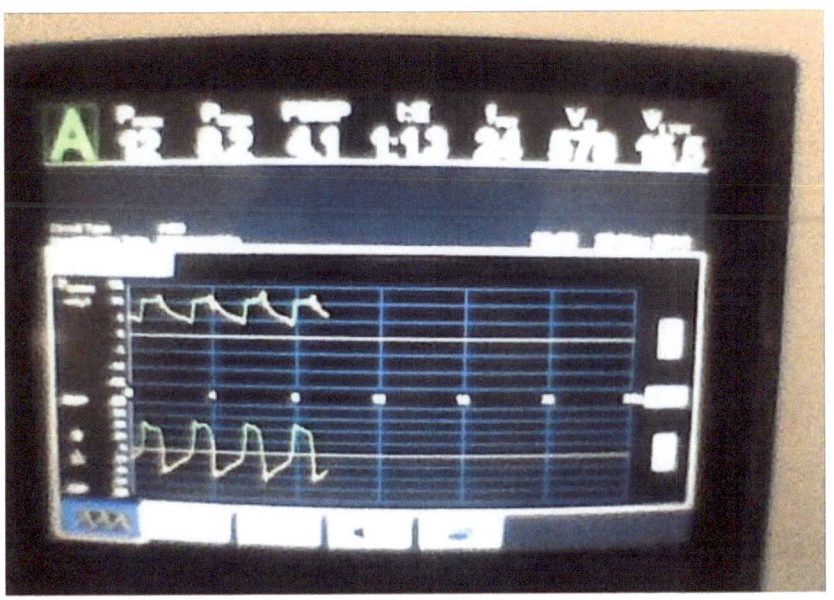

Image 110: APC in a patient with sepsis patients vigorous ventilatory drive weaned the driving pressure to 7 cmH20 (7 + 5 cmH2O of PEEP = PIP of 12 cmH2O).

Adaptive Pressure Control in a Patient with Sepsis

In patients with sepsis APC can become problematic by weaning the driving pressure prematurely due to a vigorous respiratory drive.

This patient (image 110) was a 5'-1" female patient with the following ventilator settings:
Mode: APC, Set Frequency 14, I-time 1.0 second, Set Tidal Volume 500 ml, FiO2 45%, PEEP +5 cmH2O.
Mean measured peak inspiratory pressures for 36 hours was 15 cmH2O

Initial ABG: pH 7.24, paCO2 20, PaO2 112, HCO3 8.7, BD -19 (measured minute ventilation of 16.3)

Adaptive Pressure Control in a Patient with Sepsis

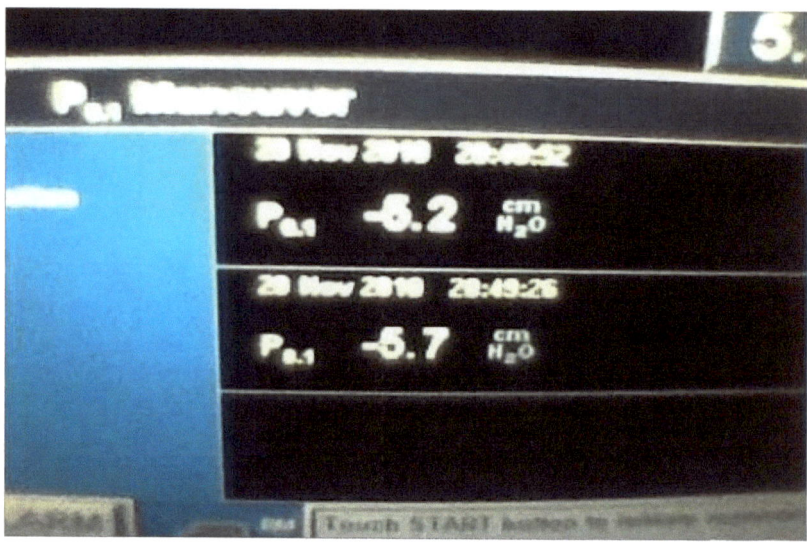

Image 111: P0.1 maneuver performed with measurements of -5.7 to -5.2 indicating large inspiratory demand.

Patient appeared very uncomfortable presenting with diaphoresis, nasal flaring, and accessory muscle use. The Airway Occlusion at 0.1 Second was assessed to evaluate the patients work load of inspiration.

The patients P0.1 measured was -5.7 to -5.2 indicating a large inspiratory effort or increased central drive. This large effort may be due to pain or agitation so the patient should be assessed further.

One way to assess if the large inspiratory effort is due to work of breathing is to increase support and reevaluate the patient & P0.1 for changes.

94

Adaptive Pressure Control in a Patient with Sepsis

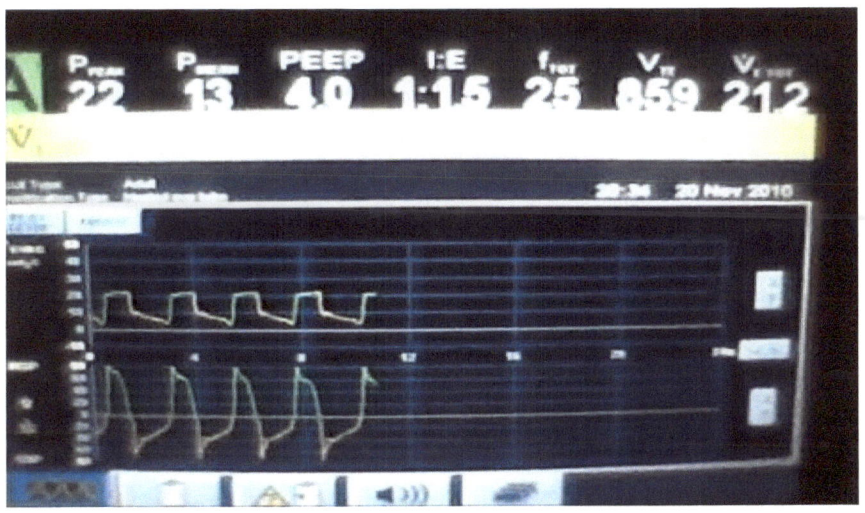

Image 112: Mode changed to PC-CMV to provide a fixed driving pressure.

Patient was switched to PC-CMV to provide a fixed driving pressure. Notice in the above image (112) how the patient's tidal volume dramatically increased, this is common with the vigorous inspiratory efforts. The tidal volumes should become smaller as the patients work of breathing decreases and the muscles off-load.

Also assess the respiratory rate, the respiratory rate should slow down if the discomfort is due to purely work of breathing (this is a key finding). If the high drive is due to agitation or pain the respiratory rate will remain the same.

Adaptive Pressure Control in a Patient with Sepsis

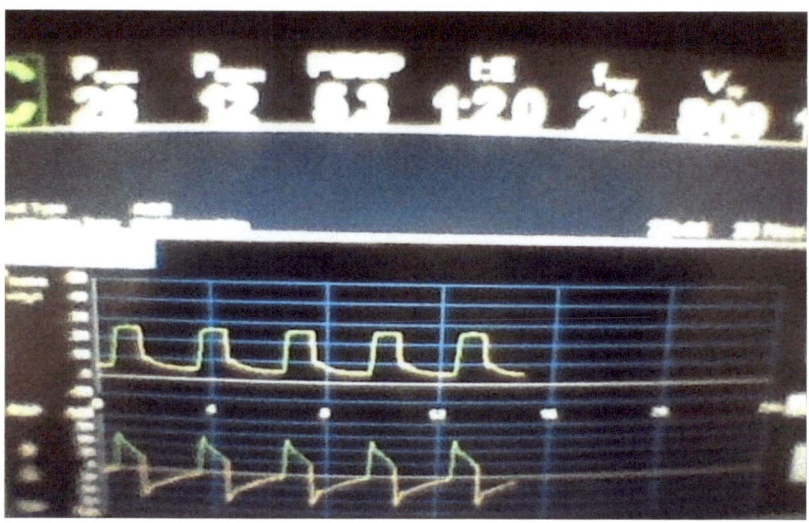

Image 113: After the patient stabilizes on PC-CMV the respiratory rate decreased, indicating distress was secondary to WOB.

The above image (112) shows the patient after stabilizing on PC-CMV. The patient's frequency decreased from a rate of 25-to-20 and tidal volume started to decrease. This indicates that the respiratory muscles are off-loading and work of breathing is decreasing. The patient's agitation was most likely due to work of breathing.

Once again evaluate P0.1 to compare if the new settings have decreased the inspiratory effort.

Adaptive Pressure Control in a Patient with Sepsis

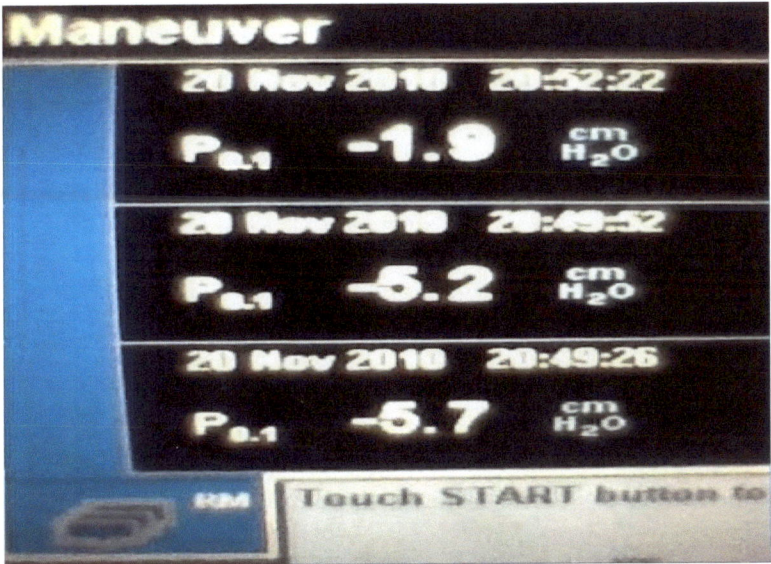

Image 114: P0.1 maneuver reevaluated, measurement went from initial reading of -5.7 to -1.9.

The Airway Occlusion at 0.1 Second was revaluated to compare the ventilator modes, settings, and patient's comfort level.
The P0.1 measurement changed dramatically in a short amount of time (~ 3 minutes). The P0.1 changed to -1.9 cmH2O associated with a low level of muscular inspiratory activity.
This demonstrates that the patient experienced a large amount of inspiratory work when ventilated with APC.

The patient remained ventilated on PC-CMV over night.

AM ABG's on PC-CMV:

pH 7.39, paCo2 19.1, paO2 210, HCO3 11.6, BD -13

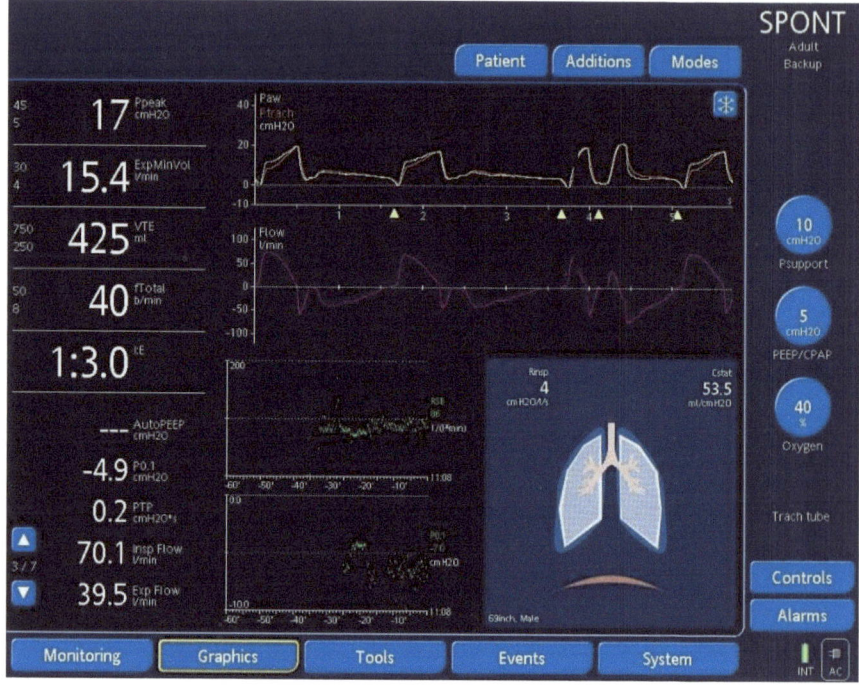

Image 115: Shows a P0.1 -4.9 indicating a high work of breathing.

Adaptive Support Ventilation Case Study

Overview: 5'-9' male patient who has failed extubation attempts & spontaneous breathing trials multiple times.

Spontaneous breathing trials (SBT) where performed using continuous spontaneous ventilation (CVS), with a PEEP of 5+ cmH2O, and a pressure support of 10 cmH2O was used to off set the imposed work of breathing (WOB) from the artificial airway and Heat Moisture Exchanger (HME).

Image 115 demonstrates the patients increased WOB during the SBT as indicated by the P0.1 of -4.9.

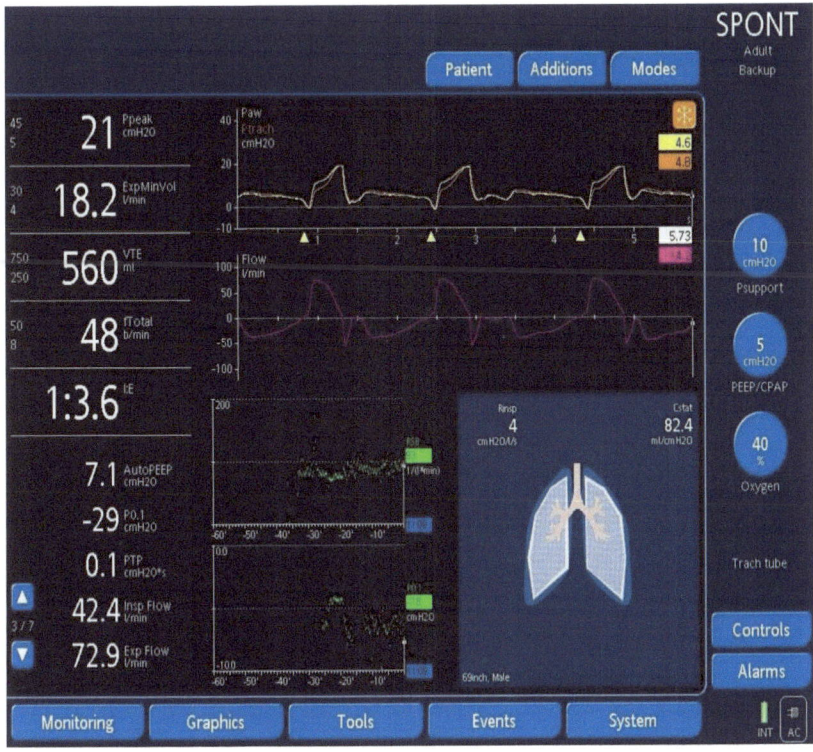

Image 116: Comparing the Rapid Shallow Breathing Index (RSBI) to the P0.1 using the trend graph.

Image 116 compares the Rapid Shallow Breathing Index (RSBI) to the P0.1, note the RSBI is less than 105 (93) which indicates potential extubation success, however the P0.1 (-7.8) indicates the patients high WOB, and that the patient would most likely wear out if ventilator support was withdrawn. P0.1 provides the clinician with additional diagnostic information.

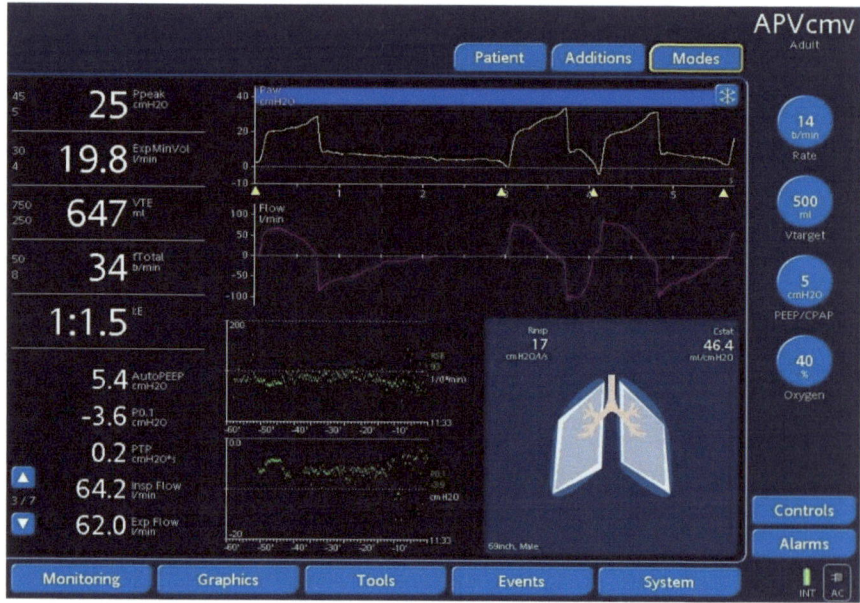

Image 117: Peak Inspiratory Pressure 25 cmH2O & P0.1 -3.6.

Rest Phase

After SBT's the patient was rested in a APC mode to off-load the respiratory muscles. To adequately off-load and rest the respiratory muscles, peak pressures of 15-20 cmH20 is generally needed to provide significant support.
This patient had a high inspiratory drive and during the rest phase APC would wean the driving pressure down, to meet the Vt target.

The images (117-119) demonstrate the weaning of the driving pressure from an initial pressure of 20 (25 PIP -5 PEEP = 20) to a driving pressure of 8 cmH20. This driving pressure of 8 (during the rest phase) is less then the pressure provided during the SBT (PS of 10 cmH2O).

Also notice the WOB increasing when the driving pressure decreases (indicated by the P0.1).
One has to consider did this patient actually get enough off-loading during the rest phase?

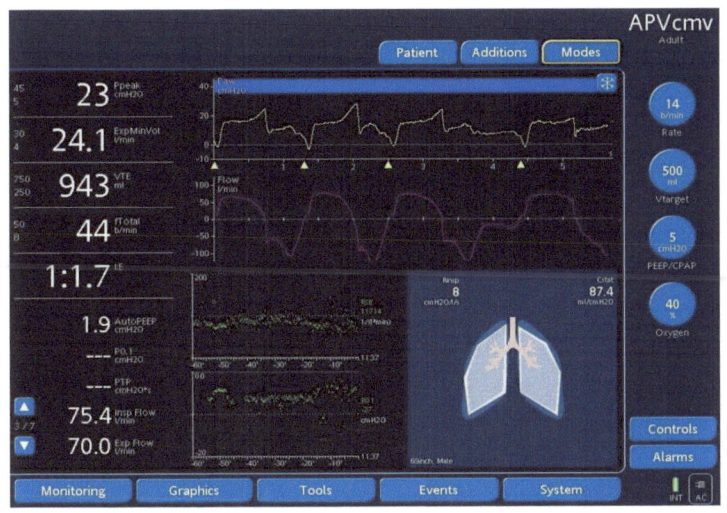

Image 118: Peak inspiratory pressure of 23 cmH2O.

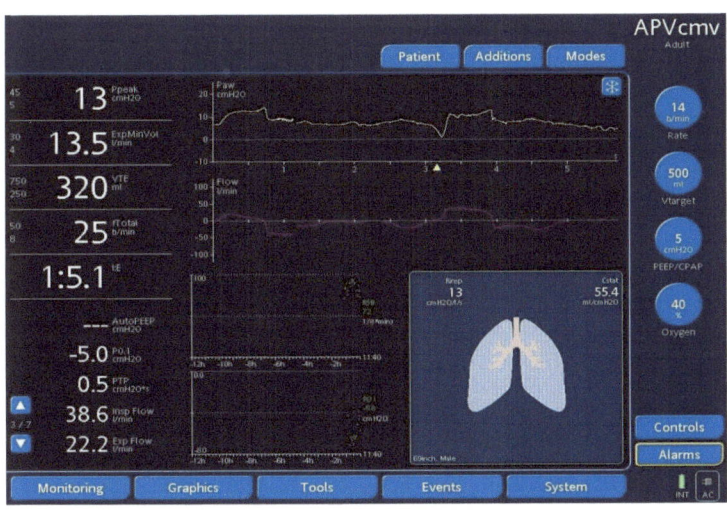

Image 119: Peak inspiratory pressure of 13 & P0.1 -5.0.

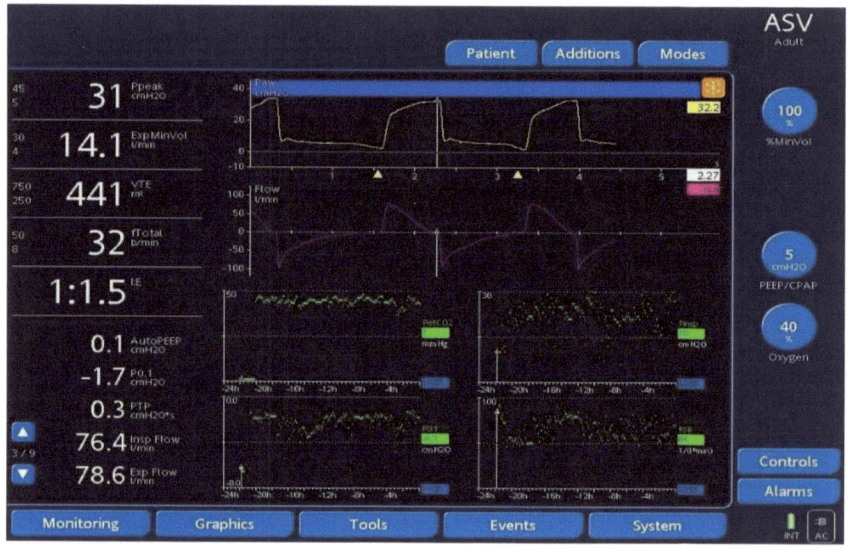

Image 120: Shows 24 hour trending with the cursor scrolled over to measurements before ASV.

ASV Initiation

The patient was switched to Adaptive Support Ventilation which is considered "Optimal Control" a modality that uses multiple mathematical models to prevent tachypnea, prevent auto-PEEP, prevent excessive dead space ventilation, prevent high pressures, maintain preset minimum minute ventilation, & fully ventilate in apnea or low respiratory drive. It also allows the patient to take control if breathing activity is within limits.

Evaluating the trending capabilities of the G5 ventilator we can review the patient's respiratory status over a period of 1, 12, or 24 hours. In this twenty-four hour view four parameters were trended (EtCO2, Pinsp, P0.1, & RSBI). The screen is frozen & the arrow is scrolled back when patient was on an APC mode, showing lower driving pressures (10cmH2O) and a higher WOB (P0.1 -6.3).

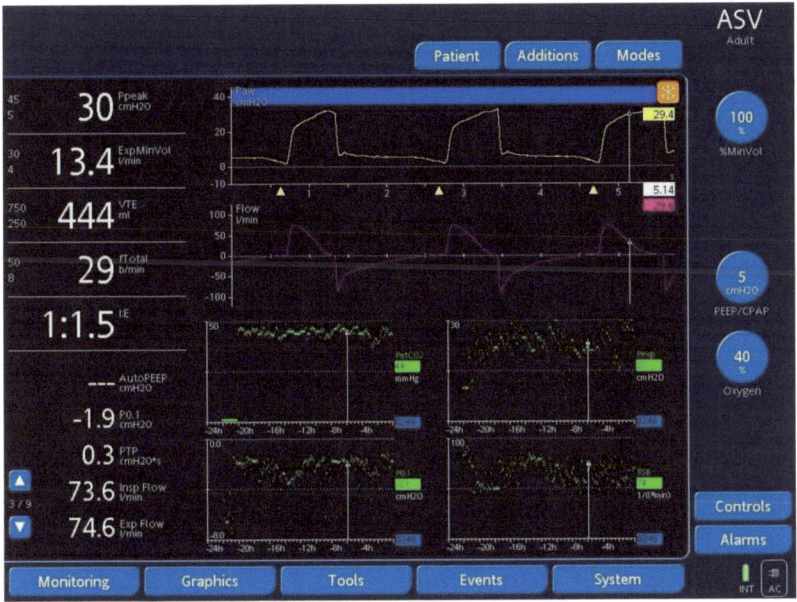

Image 121: Shows 24 hour trending with the cursor scrolled over to measurements ~ 15 hours initiation.

Reviewing the twenty-four hour trends, one notices that the driving pressure rarely dropped below the mid-twenties. The mathematical model prevented the ventilator from titrating the pressure down which would have resulted in excessive dead-space ventilation, increased WOB, and respiratory muscle fatigue. This review of trends confirms that when the patient was in an APC mode the premature decreasing of driving pressure most likely resulted in further respiratory muscle fatigue & inappropriate off-loading of respiratory muscles during the patients rest phase.

103

References

Trigger Asynchronies

[1] Epstein, S. (2011). How Often Does Patient-Ventilator Asynchrony Occur & What are the Consequences? *Respiratory Care*. 56 (1).

[2] Lotti, G. Brashi, A. Measurements of Respiratory Mechanics During Mechanical Ventilation. Rhuzuns, Switzerland. 1999: 103-113.

[3] Younes,M. (circa 2006). Lecture on PAV+. Covidien Healthcare. Boulder, Co.

[4] Sassoon, C. (2011). Triggering of the Ventilator in Patient-Ventilator Interactions. *Respiratory Care*. 56 (1):39-46.

[5] Kacmarek, R. (2011). Proportional Assist Ventilation And Neurally Adjusted Ventilatory Assist. *Respiratory Care*. 56 (2): 140-144.

[6] Chatburn, R. (2007). Classification of Ventilator Modes: Update and Proposal for Implementation. *Respiratory Care*. 52 (92): 311-312.

Flow Asynchronies

[7] Esteban et. Al. (2008). *American Journal of Respiratory Care*. 177:170-177.

[8] Levine, S. et. Al. (2008). Rapid Disuse Atrophy of Diaphragm Fibers in Mechanically Ventilated Humans. *New England Journal of Medicine*. 358 (13): 1327-1425.

[9] Kallet, R. et. Al. (2005). Work of Breathing During Lung-Protective Ventilation in Patients with Acute Lung Injury and Acute Respiratory Distress Syndrome: a Comparison Between Volume and Pressure Regulated Breathing Modes. *Respiratory Care*. 50 (12): 1622-1631.

[10] Steinburg, K. & Kacmarek, R. (2007). Should Tidal Volume be 6 ml/kg Predicted Body Weight in Virtually all Patients with Acute Respiratory Failure? *Respiratory Care*. 52 (5): 556.

[11] Nilsestuen, J. & Hargett, K. (2005). Using Ventilator Graphics to Identify Patient-Ventilator Asynchrony. *Respiratory Care*. 50 (2): 202-231.

[12] Branson, R. (2011). Patient-Ventilator Interaction: the Last 40 Years. *Respiratory Care*. 56 (1): 19-23.

[13] Marini, J et. Al (1989). Determinants and limits of Pressure-Preset Ventilation: a Mathematical Model of Pressure Control. *Journal of Applied Physiology*. 67 (3): 1081-1092.

Cycling Asynchronies

[14] Gentile, M. (2011). Cycling of the Mechanical Ventilator Breath. *Respiratory Care*. 56 (1).

References

Expiratory Asynchronies

[14] Gentile, M. (2011). Cycling of the Mechanical Ventilator Breath. *Respiratory Care.* 56 (1).

Adaptive Pressure Control

[15] Jaecklin, T et. Al (2007). Volume-Targeted Modes of Modern Neonatal Ventilators: How Stable is the Delivered Tidal Volume? *Intensive Care Medicine.* 33 (2).

Adaptive Support Ventilation

[16] Chatburn, R. & Mireles, E. (2011). Closed-Loop Control of Mechanical Ventilation: Description and Classification of Targeting Schemes. *Respiratory Care.* 56 (1).
[17] (2006). Adaptive Support Ventilation User's Guide. Hamilton Medical AG. Bonaduz, Swtizerland.